Practical Tips For
INFERTILITY MANAGEMENT

Practical Tips For
INFERTILITY MANAGEMENT

"THE RAINBOW PROTOCOLS"

Series Editor
Jaideep Malhotra MBBS MD FICOG

Editorial Board
**Narendra Malhotra, Diksha Goswami,
Shally Gupta, Neharika Malhotra Bora,
Keshav Malhotra, Pramod Bajaj,
Rishabh Bora, Ajay Srivastava,
Shilpa Marwah, Manpreet Kaur,
Bhagwan Singh, Richa Sharma,
Richa Saxena, Shobhna Arora**

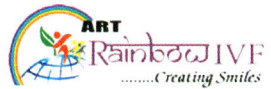

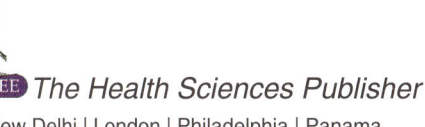

The Health Sciences Publisher
New Delhi | London | Philadelphia | Panama

Jaypee Brothers Medical Publishers (P) Ltd

Headquarters

Jaypee Brothers Medical Publishers (P) Ltd
4838/24, Ansari Road, Daryaganj
New Delhi 110 002, India
Phone: +91-11-43574357
Fax: +91-11-43574314
Email: jaypee@jaypeebrothers.com

Overseas Offices

J.P. Medical Ltd
83 Victoria Street, London
SW1H 0HW (UK)
Phone: +44 20 3170 8910
Fax: +44 (0)20 3008 6180
Email: info@jpmedpub.com

Jaypee Medical Inc
The Bourse
111 South Independence Mall East
Suite 835, Philadelphia, PA 19106, USA
Phone: +1 267-519-9789
Email: jpmed.us@gmail.com

Jaypee Brothers Medical Publishers (P) Ltd
Bhotahity, Kathmandu, Nepal
Phone: +977-9741283608
Email: kathmandu@jaypeebrothers.com

Jaypee-Highlights Medical Publishers Inc
City of Knowledge, Bld. 237, Clayton
Panama City, Panama
Phone: +1 507-301-0496
Fax: +1 507-301-0499
Email: cservice@jphmedical.com

Jaypee Brothers Medical Publishers (P) Ltd
17/1-B Babar Road, Block-B, Shaymali
Mohammadpur, Dhaka-1207
Bangladesh
Mobile: +08801912003485
Email: jaypeedhaka@gmail.com

Website: www.jaypeebrothers.com
Website: www.jaypeedigital.com

© 2016, Jaypee Brothers Medical Publishers

The views and opinions expressed in this book are solely those of the original contributor(s)/author(s) and do not necessarily represent those of editor(s) of the book.

All rights reserved. No part of this publication may be reproduced, stored or transmitted in any form or by any means, electronic, mechanical, photocopying, recording or otherwise, without the prior permission in writing of the publishers.

All brand names and product names used in this book are trade names, service marks, trademarks or registered trademarks of their respective owners. The publisher is not associated with any product or vendor mentioned in this book.

Medical knowledge and practice change constantly. This book is designed to provide accurate, authoritative information about the subject matter in question. However, readers are advised to check the most current information available on procedures included and check information from the manufacturer of each product to be administered, to verify the recommended dose, formula, method and duration of administration, adverse effects and contraindications. It is the responsibility of the practitioner to take all appropriate safety precautions. Neither the publisher nor the author(s)/editor(s) assume any liability for any injury and/or damage to persons or property arising from or related to use of material in this book.

This book is sold on the understanding that the publisher is not engaged in providing professional medical services. If such advice or services are required, the services of a competent medical professional should be sought.

Every effort has been made where necessary to contact holders of copyright to obtain permission to reproduce copyright material. If any have been inadvertently overlooked, the publisher will be pleased to make the necessary arrangements at the first opportunity.

Inquiries for bulk sales may be solicited at: jaypee@jaypeebrothers.com

Practical Tips for Infertility Management

First Edition: **2016**

ISBN 978-93-5152-883-8

Printed at Sanat Printers

Dedication

This effort of ours to simplify Infertility Management is dedicated to Late Dr. Mrs. Prabha Malhotra and to my late parents Ms & Mr. H. S. Bindra. Parents were the one's who made sure that I got educated and Late. Dr. Prabha Malhotra was the one who taught us patient care.

Salute to them

Preface

Infertility is a major health problem today. Almost 15% couples are infertile, unable to conceive within year of married life. An absolute 30 million infertile couples (equal to population of Australia and more than the population of many countries) live in India.

Today the need is to manage infertility step wise with an active management protocol. The idea is not to waste patient's time, money and precious ovarian reserve. Active management according to age and ovarian reserve has been described as algorithms in this manual.

Patient counseling and couple interview with proper preconceptional nutritional advise and supplementations is equally if not more important as actual treatment.

This manual aims to describe practical tips for the practitioners and, we hope, will help the doctors.

Happy reading

Jaideep Malhotra

Contents

1. Introduction to the Problem — 1
2. An Approach to Infertility — 4
3. Infertility: FAQs — 96
   Appendix — *119*
   Index — *127*

Introduction to the Problem

Chapter 1

- 15% of all couples have infertility
- 40% is female factor
- 40% is male factor
- 20% is unexplained
- Natural fecundity is 20% each cycle, 50% at 3 months and 85% at 12 months
- Older the women more the infertility. 90% of women will not conceive at >40 years of age
- Males also show decreased fertility potential with age
- Frequency of intercourse affects fertility
- Occupational hazards influence fertility potential
- Previous contraception use also has an influence
- Stress plays an important role

Figure 1.1 showing various factors playing a role in infertility control.

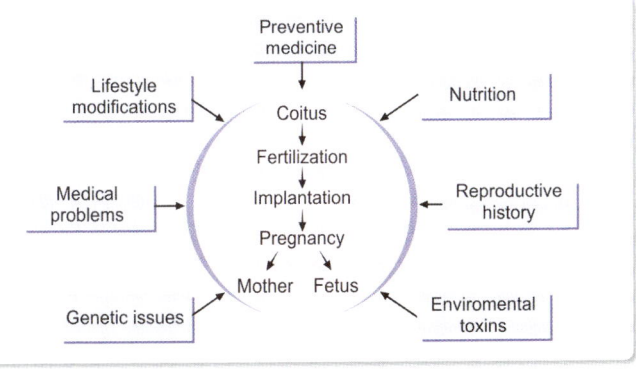

Fig. 1.1: Factors in infertility control

Pathway of Conception (Fig. 1.2)

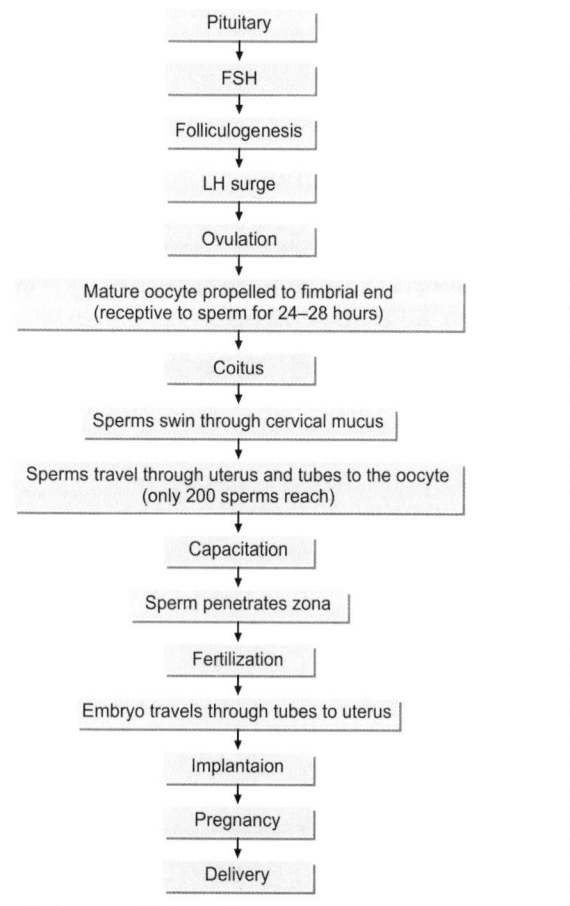

Fig. 1.2: Pathway of conception

Embryo Development and Implantation (Fig. 1.3)

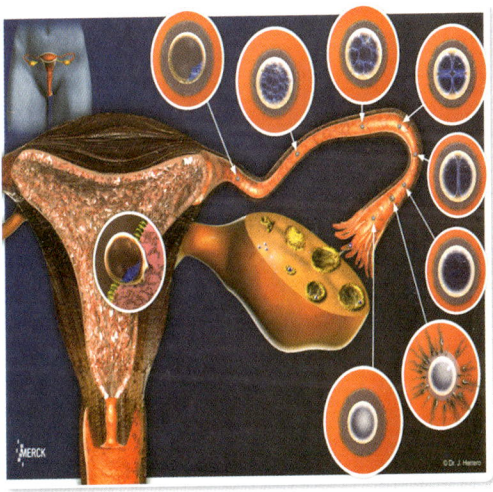

Fig. 1.3: Embryo development and implantation

An Approach to Infertility

2
Chapter

- ❑ Evaluation work up
- ❑ Management

Evaluation

The infertile couple should be investigated after 1 year of regular unprotected intercourse with adequate frequency. The interval is however shortened to 6 months after the age of 35 years of the woman and 40 years of man.

Both the partners should come for the initial interview and should be evaluated and treated together, as infertility is not the disease of only the woman. The causes with approximate percentages are shown in **Figure 2.1**.

Cause	%
Male	35–40
Female	40
Combined	10
Idiopathic	10

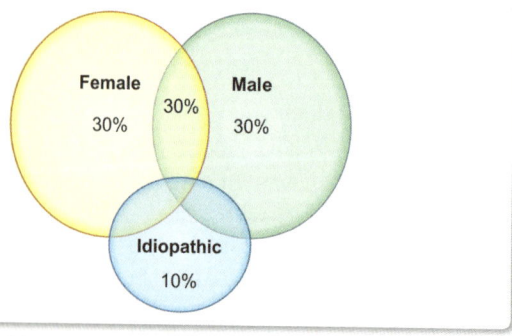

Fig. 2.1: Male, female and idiopathic causes of infertility

An Approach to Infertility

Preconception Advice and Counseling

- Medical check-up for fitness
- Medications
- Exposure to occupational and environmental toxins
- Pre-pregnant health evaluation
- Evaluation of medical, social, genetic, environmental and occupational factors
- Advice and counseling
- Life style habits
- Not to use tobacco, alcohol and other recreational drugs
- Sexual habits and lubricant use counseling
- Good nutrition and exercises, including yoga and back massage
- Reduction of body weight for obese patients
- Vitamin, antioxidants, methylating agent supplementations
- Herbal remedies some herbal medicines are detrimental to sperm and oocytes like St. John's Wort, Echinacea purpura and Ginkgo biloba while most of them are beneficial
- Pre-pregnant low dose Aspirin (for older women?)
- Screening for blood disorders in couple and vaccination against Rubella
- Treatment and control of diabetes, thyroid, hyperprolactenemia and other diseases
- Pap's smear and routine breast examination and mammography
- Genetic counselling and screening

Counseling Check List

- Interview with couple together   Yes/No
- Separate interview with female   Yes/No
- Separate interview with male   Yes/No
- All above points discussed   Yes/No
- All treatment modalities discussed   Yes/No
  (Including 3rd party)

- ❏ Costs and expenses discussed   Yes/No
- ❏ Option of adoption discussed   Yes/No

Causes of Infertility (Fig. 2.2)

- ❏ Male factor   35–40%
- ❏ Female factor   40%
  - Ovulatory   20–40%
  - Tubal   20–40%
  - Endometriosis   10%
  - Advanced age   18–50%
  - Luteal phase defects   <10%
  - Uterine and cervical facts   10%
  - Fibroids   2–3%
- ❏ Unexplained   10–15%
- ❏ Combination   10–20%

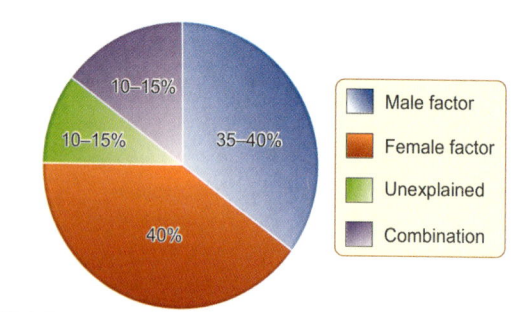

Fig. 2.2: Factors in infertility (%)

Male Factors

1. Ejaculatory factors
- ❏ Spinal cord injury
- ❏ Impotence
- ❏ Retrograde ejaculation
- ❏ Premature ejaculation

An Approach to Infertility

2. Anatomical factors (Fig. 2.3)
- Cryptorchidism
- Hypospadias
- Epispadias
- Varicocele
- Cogenital absence of Vas

3. Sperm factors (Figs 2.4 to 2.6)
- Oligozoospermia

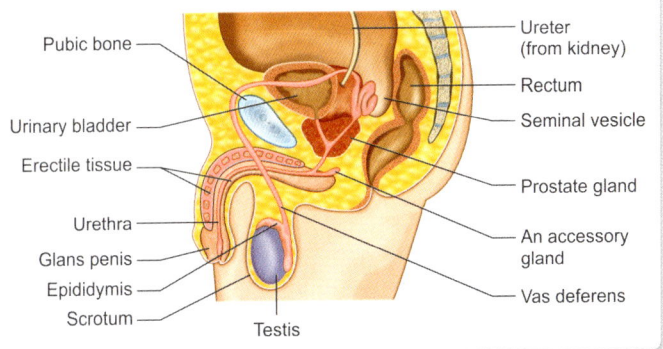

Fig. 2.3: Male reproductive system

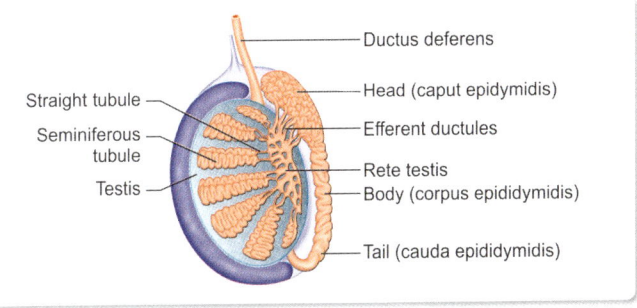

Fig. 2.4: Section of testis

8 Practical Tips for Infertility Management

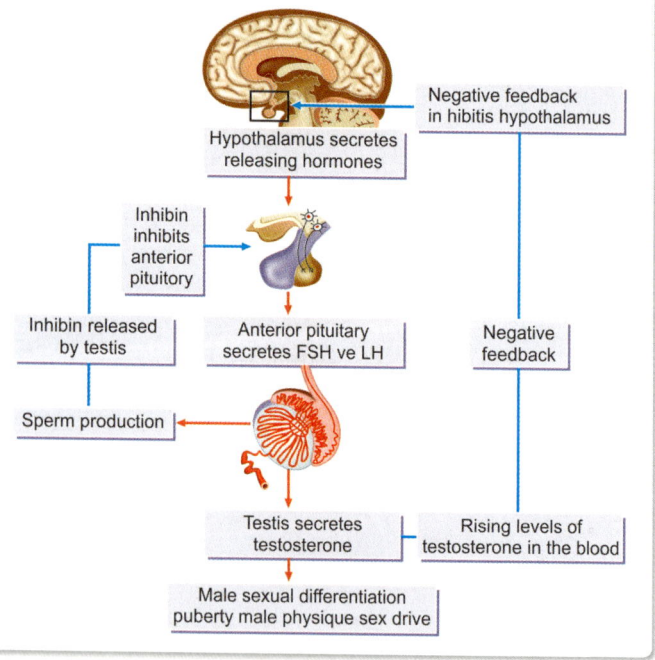

Fig. 2.5: Hormonal circuit in males

- Asthenooligozoospermia
- Teratozoospermia
- Oligoasthenozoospermia
- Necrozoospermia

4. Immunological infertility
- ASA in serum
- ASA in seminal fluid
- Clumping of sperms

5. Viscous semen

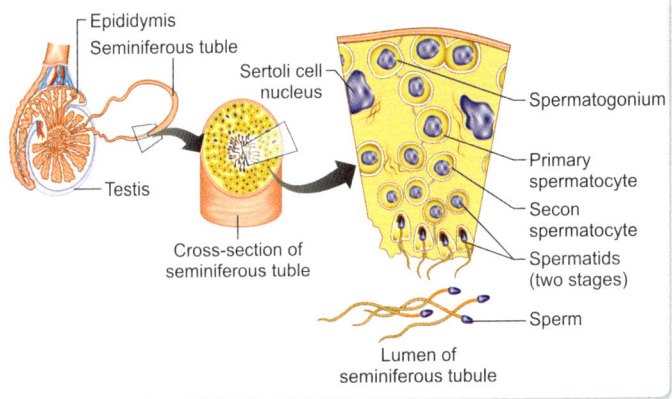

Fig. 2.6: Spermatogenesis in testis

6. Genetic factors
- 47, XXY
- 46, XY-mosaic
- Azoospermic

7. Endocrine factors
- Thyroid dysfunction
- Cushing disease
- Acromegaly
- Pituitary tumor

8. Infective factor
- Tuberculosis
- Gonorrhea
- Chlamydia

9. Other factors
- Environmental factors
- Medication

- Trauma
- Psycological

Female Anatomy and Physiology

It is important to understand female external and internal reproductive system **(Figs 2.7 and 2.8)**.

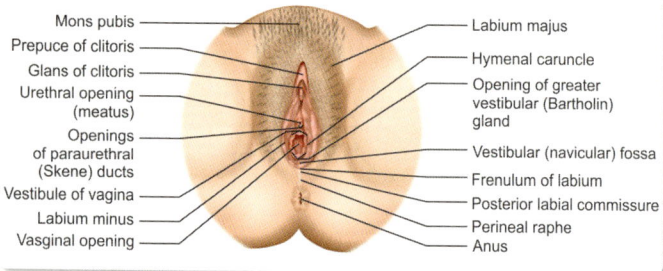

Fig. 2.7: External genitalia of female

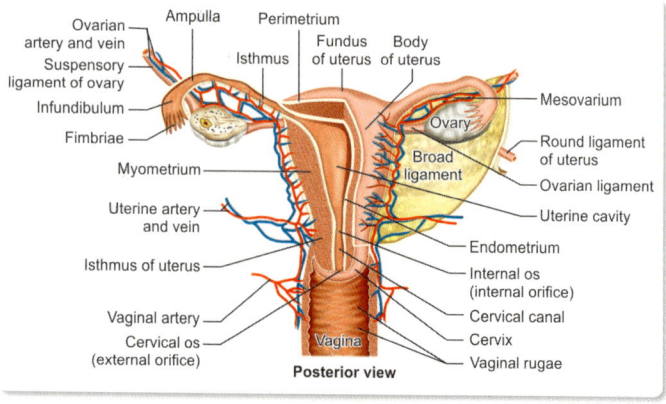

Fig. 2.8A: Female reproductive system

An Approach to Infertility 11

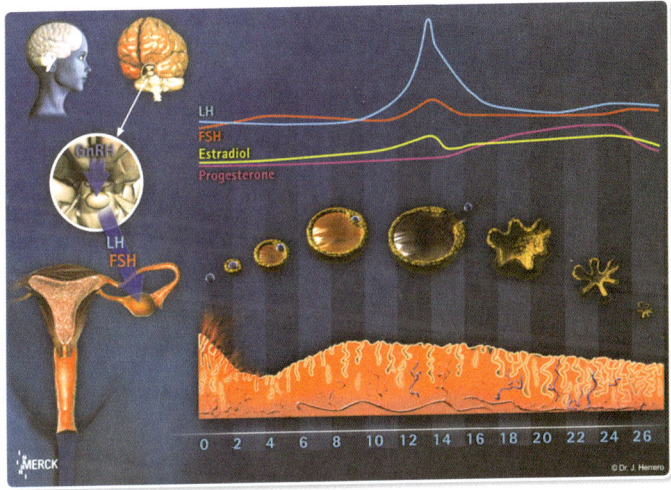

Fig. 2.8B: Menstrual cycle

Also a good understanding for female physiology and hypothalamic-pituitary-ovarian-endometrial-peripheral axis is needed **(Fig. 2.8)**.

Cyclical changes in a menstrual cycle are important **(Figs 2.9 and 2.10)**.

Causes Organwise (Female)

a. Hypothalamus **(Figs 2.10 and 2.11)**
   – Weight
   – Exercise
   – Polycystic ovarian syndrome (PCOS)
   – Systemic diseases (Liver/Kidney)
   – Kallmann's syndrome
b. Pituitary gland **(Fig. 2.11)**
   – Hyperprolactinemia

12 Practical Tips for Infertility Management

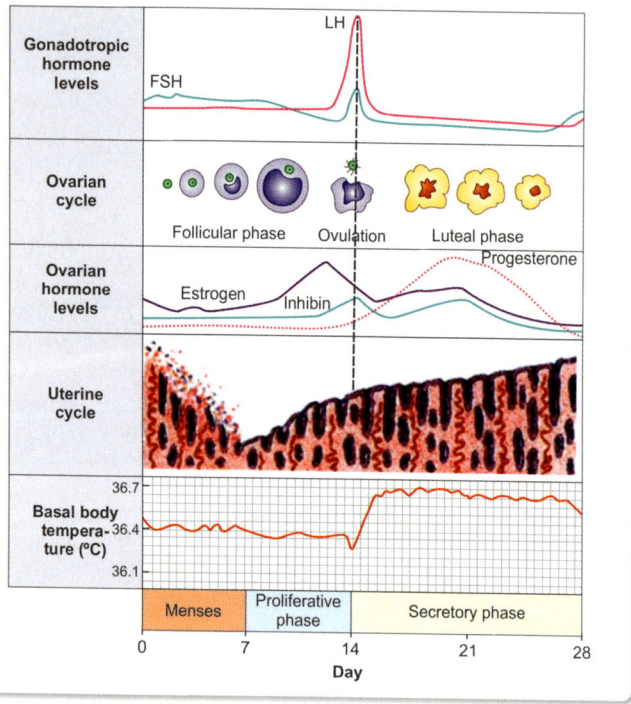

Fig. 2.9: Overview of follicular growth and hormonal regulation

- Hypothyriodism
- Sheehan's syndrome
- Hypo-hypo syndrome
c. Ovary
    - Premature ovarian failure (POF)
    - Luteinized unruptured follicle (LUF)
    - PCOS **(Figs 2.12 and 2.13)**

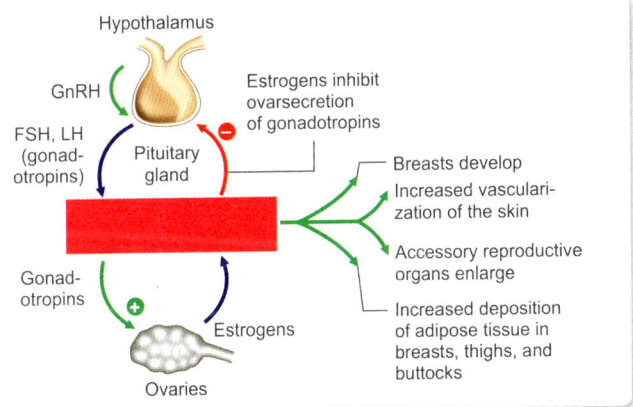

Fig. 2.10: Hormonal regulation in females

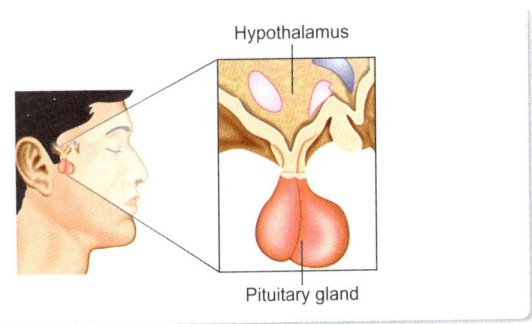

Fig. 2.11: Hypothalmus and pituitary

- Luteal phase defects (LPD)
- Oligo and anovulation
d. Fallopian tubes
   - Blocked (**Fig. 2.14**)

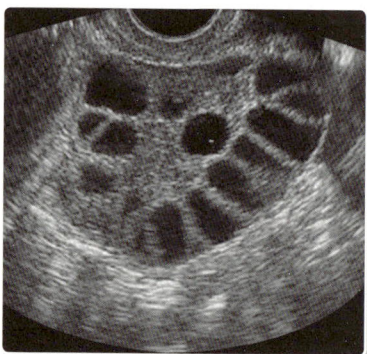

Fig. 2.12: PCOS ovaries

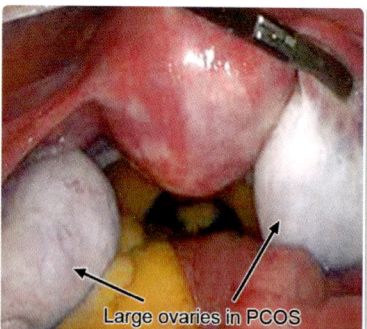

Fig. 2.13: PCOS ovaries

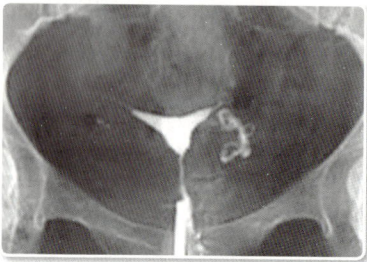

Fig. 2.14: One blocked fallopian tube

An Approach to Infertility 15

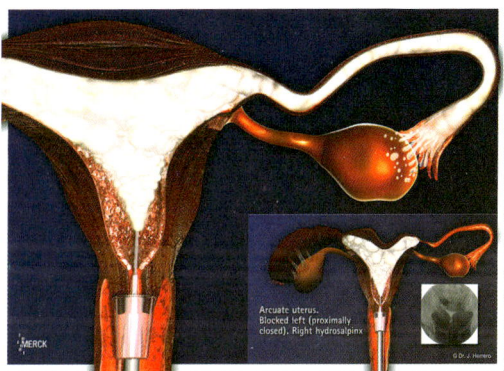

Fig. 2.15: Hysterosalpingography

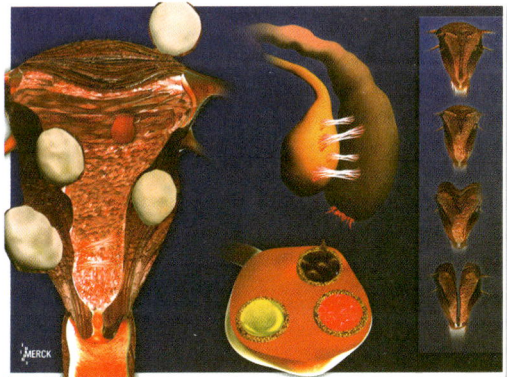

Fig. 2.16: Uterine, ovarian and tubal abnormalities

- Infections (PID)
- Tuberculosis
e. Uterus **(Figs 2.15 and 2.16)**
    - Asherman's syndrome
    - Fibroids

- Polyps
- Müllerian defects

f. Cervix **(Figs 2.17 to 2.19)**
   - Poor cervical mucous
   - Cervicitis **(Fig. 2.17)**
   - Cervical stenosis
g. Immunological factors
   - ASA in serum
   - ASA in cervix mucus
h. Sexual dysfunction
i. Others
   - Douching
   - Smoking
j. Unexplained factors
   - Fertilization defects
   - Infertility >2 years with
   - Normal HSG/Lap
   - Normal hormonal levels
   - Negative ASA
   - ± Hysteroscopy
   - ± Follicular/endo growth on USG

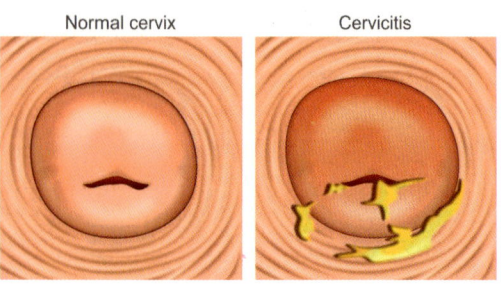

Fig. 2.17: Cervix and cervicitis

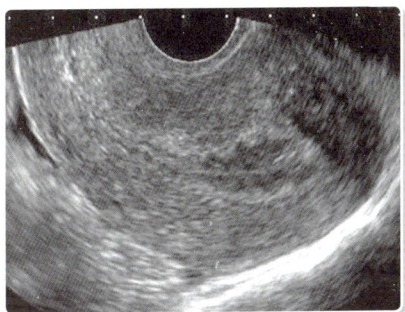

Fig. 2.18: USG evaluation of cervix

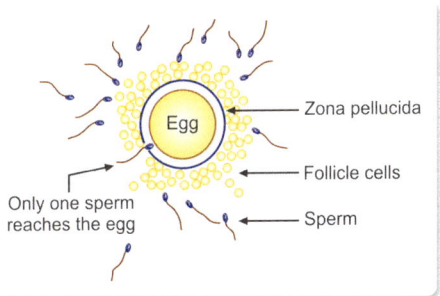

Fig. 2.19: Fertilization process

Typical Sequence of Infertility Work-up

Step I

Initial Interview and Examination **(Figs 2.20 and 2.21)**

- Both partners should be present
- History and general physical examination of both partners
- Outline tests and investigations
- Answer questions
- Tests for ureaplasma and chlymadia.

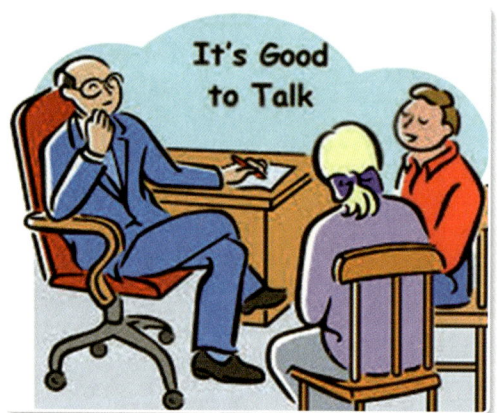

Fig. 2.20: Patient counselling

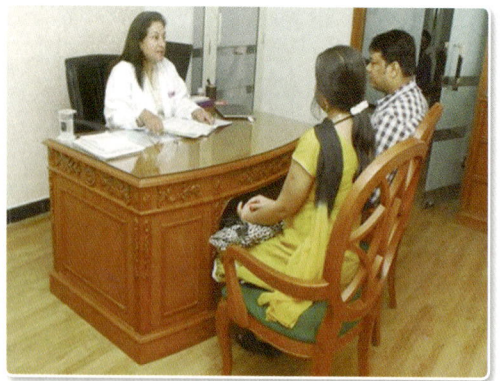

Fig. 2.21: Dr Jaideep consulting with patient

Step II

Laboratory Evaluations **(Figs 2.22 and 2.23)**

MEN
Semen analysis (after suitable abstinence) **(Figs 2.24 to 2.30)**

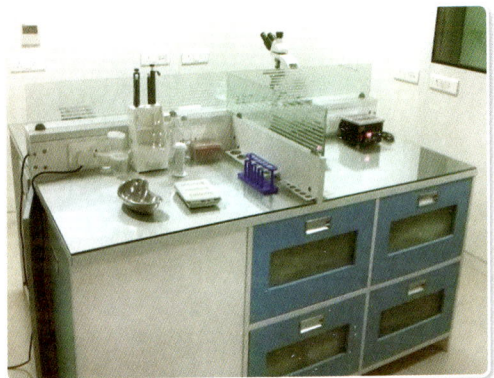

Fig. 2.22: Andrology (semenology) lab

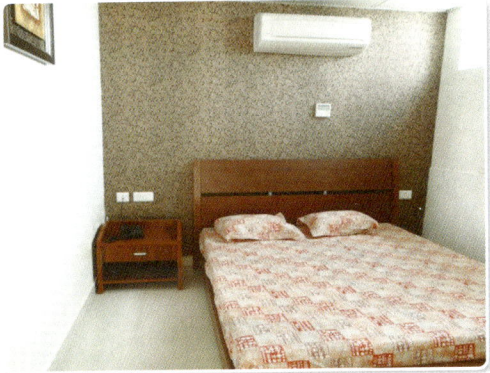

Fig. 2.23: Semen collection room

WOMEN (Beginning with next menstruation)
- Basal body temperature (BBT) **(Fig. 2.31)**
- Ovulation detection kit **(Fig. 2.32)**
- Hormone assays is indicated
- Hysterosalpingography/sonosalpigography **(Fig. 2.33)**

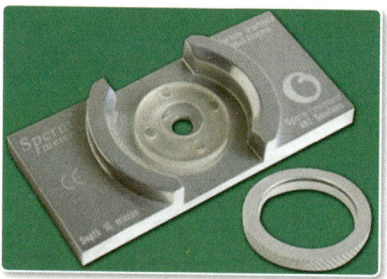

Fig. 2.24: Sperm counting chamber

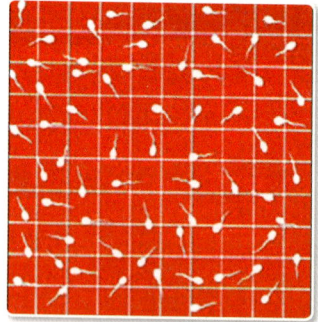

Fig. 2.25: Normal sperm count

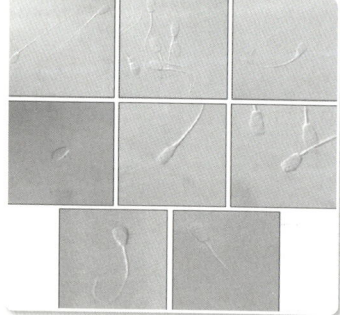

Fig. 2.26: Low sperm count

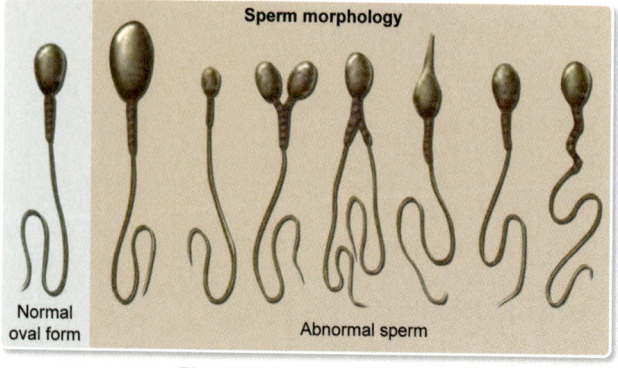

Fig. 2.27: Abnormal sperms

An Approach to Infertility

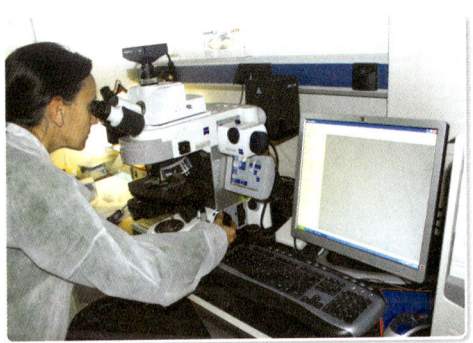

Fig. 2.28: CASA machine

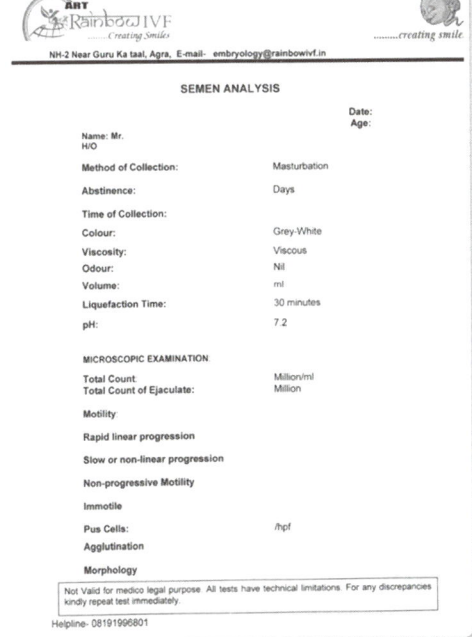

Fig. 2.29: Semen analysis report

WHO criteria for normal sperm

	5th edition	4th edition
Volume (m/s)	1.5	2.0
Total sperm (millions in ejac)	39	40
Sperm conc. (millions per ml)	15	20
Total motility	40	50
% Normal forms	4	(14)

Fig. 2.30: WHO 2012 normal semen parameters

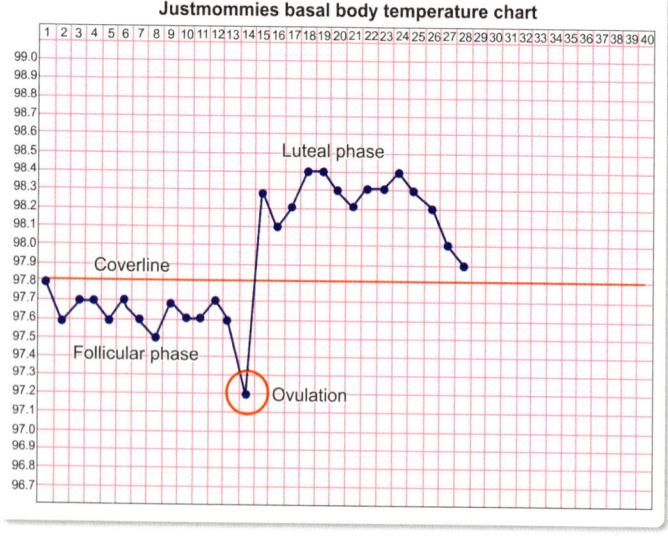

Fig. 2.31: BBT chart

- Follicular ultrasonography **(Figs 2.34 to 2.38)**
- Post coital test
- For ammenorhea/oligomenorrhea begin with hormone studies
- After induction of ovulation proceed to above studies.

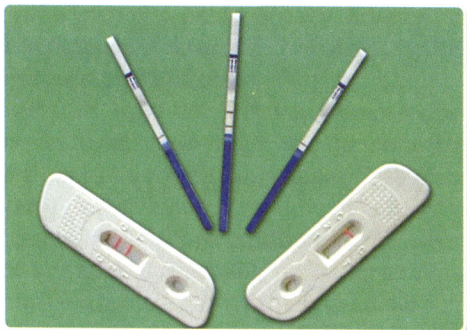

Fig. 2.32: Ovulation detection kits

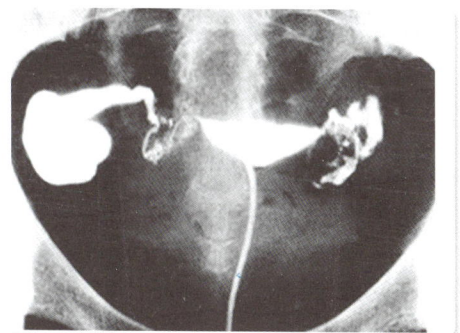

Fig. 2.33: Hysterosalpingography

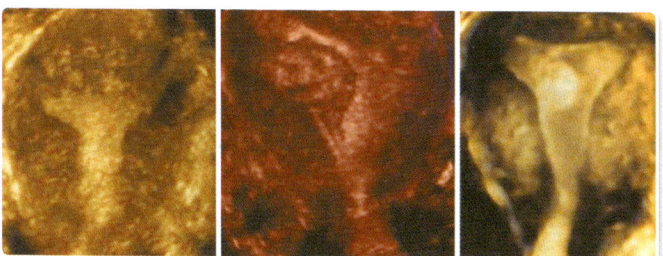

Fig. 2.34: Day 2 baseline scan

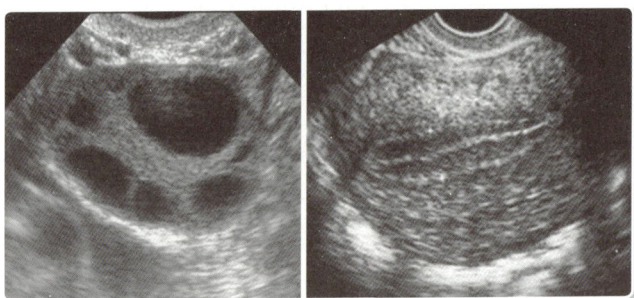

Fig. 2.35: Day 6 scan follicle and endometrium

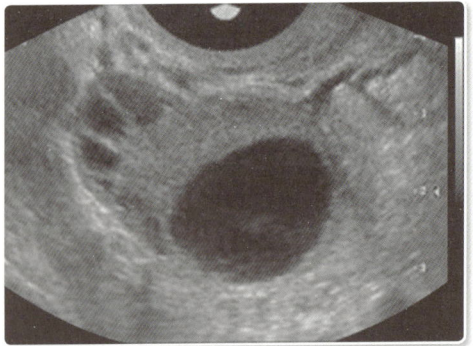

Fig. 2.36: Day 12 scan (pre-ovulatory)

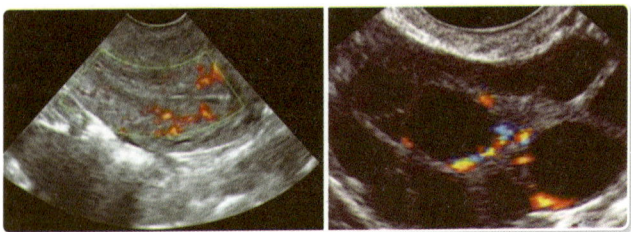

Fig. 2.37: Color Doppler in follicles and endometrium

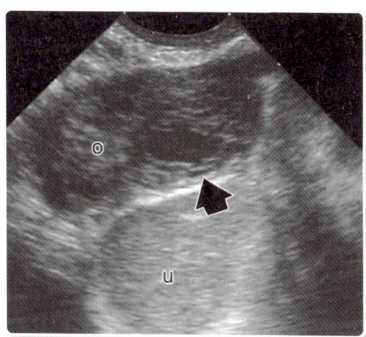

Fig. 2.38: Post-ovulatory scan

Step III

Specialized Test

Men
- Abnormal semen analysis **(see Fig. 2.27)**
- Serum FSH, LH, TSH, testosterone
- Fructose content of semen
- Prostatic massage and culture sensitivity of the fluid

Women
- Hysterosalpingogram or contrast sonography 3D Hycosy
- Laparoscopy and hysteroscopy
- Endometrial biopsy for tuberculosis

Step IV

Continue Investigations Based on Positive Findings

Men
- Testicular biopsy **(Figs 2.39 and 2.40)**
- Sex chromatin study
- Immunological tests

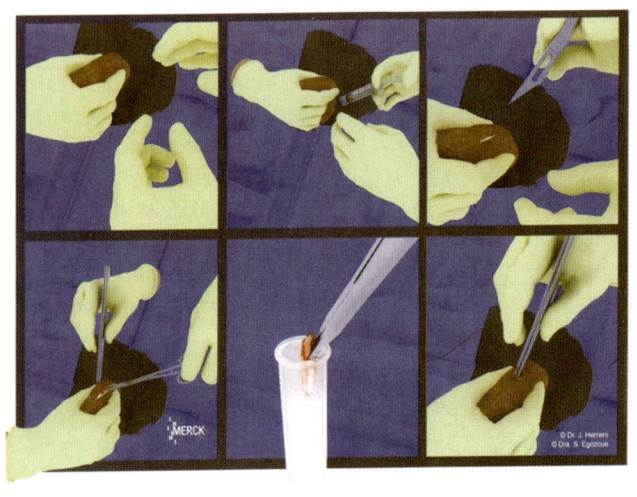

Fig. 2.39: Testicular biopsy

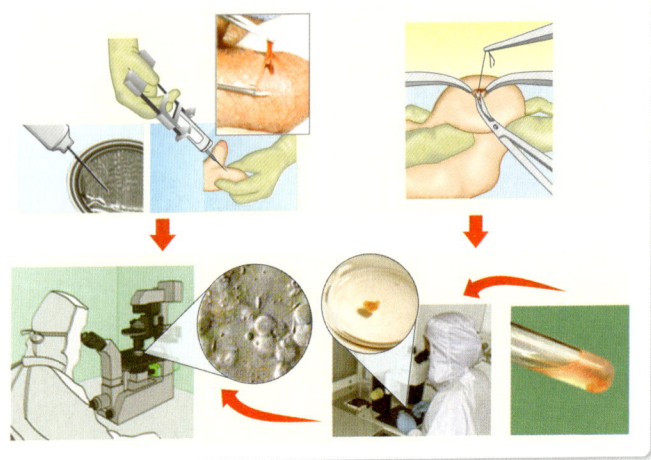

Fig. 2.40A: TESA

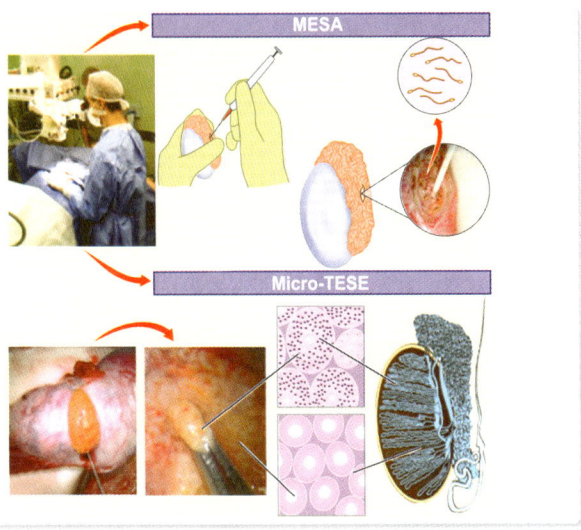

Fig. 2.40B: MESA

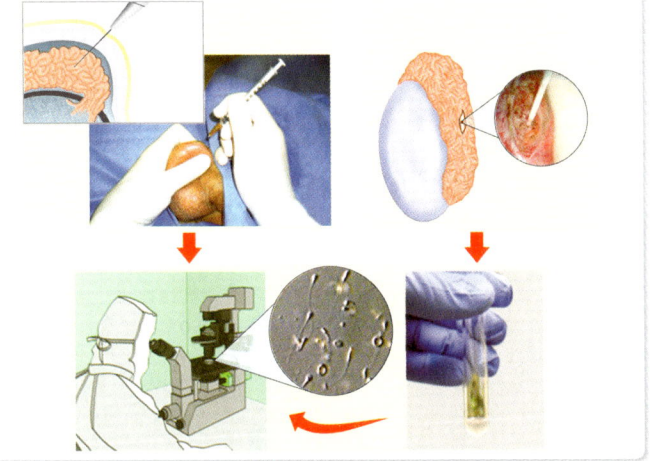

Fig. 2.40C: PESA

Women
- Hysteroscopy and laparoscopy for pelvic or after pathology
- Anti-sperm antibody test
- CT scan and MRI for tumors of pituitary/hypothalamus/adrenal glands

Clinical Approach to Investigation

Male

History
- Age
- Duration of marriage
- History of proven fertility if any
- General medical history especially of
- Sexually transmitted disease and treatment taken, of
- Mumps orchitis after puberty, history of
- Diabetes mellitus, tuberculosis
- Relevant surgery done, e.g. herniorrhaphy, operation on testis or any other genital operation
- Occupational history toward exposure to radiation/excessive heat
- Sexual history—frequency of intercourse, full penetration of penis inside the vagina, orgasm at the right time (premature ejaculation)
- Social habits, heavy smoking, alcohol and drug abuse.

Examination
- General physical examination
- Reproductive system examination
- Inspection and palpation of genitalia
- Presence of varicocele **(Fig. 2.41)**

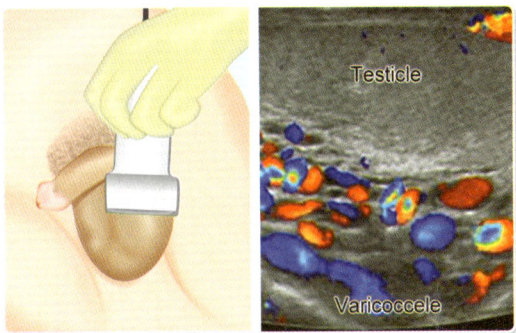

Fig. 2.41: USG of varicocele

Special Investigation
- Routine investigations
- Routine blood examination
    - Complete urine examination
    - CBC, blood group
    - B. Sugar
        - Fasting
        - Post-prandial
    - VDRL
    - HpB, HCV, HIV
    - TSH, PRL

Summary of infertility checklist for male and female is given in **Figure 2.42**.

Seminal fluid analysis collected by masturbation into a clean wide mouthed bottle preferably in the laboratory with a prior abstinence for 2 days. A normal sperminogram is tabulated in **Figure 2.43**.

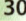 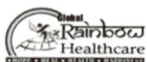 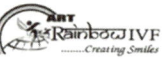

NH-2, Near Guru Ka Taal, Agra, Ph.: +91 - 0562-2600531-536
E-mail : ivf@rainbowhospitals.org, Web : www.rainbowivf.in

PRE I.V.F. EVALUATION TESTS & INVESTIGATIONS

INFERTILITY PANEL   Date : ....

Name : ....

WIFE

A. Routine Tests
1. Hb+Hb Th
2. TLC/DLC/Platelets/GBP
3. Bl Group ABO/Rh
4. Bl Sugar F/R/PP
   Glucose Tolerance Test
5. VDRL
6. HIV
7. HpB
8. HpC (HCV)
9. Urine R/M
10. Blood Urea
11. S. Creatine
12. L.F.T.
13. Others

B. Day 2 of Menstrual Cycle Tests
FSH/LH/PRL/TSH/E2/DHEAS
A.M.H.

C. Special Investigations
TORCH Profile
APLA Profile
Karyotyping
3-D USG (TVS) for Cavity
Mock E.T.
Cx Swab $\langle^C_S$ & PAP's Smear
Vaginal Swab for BV & Chlamydia
Diagnostic Hysteroscopy

D. Autogen / RSA-BOH Panel

P.T.O.

HUSBAND

A. Routine Tests
1. Hb+Hb Th
2. TLC/DLC/Platelets/GBP
3. Bl Group ABO/Rh
4. Bl Sugar F/R/PP
   Glucose Tolerance Test
5. VDRL
6. HIV
7. HpB / HpC
8. Urine R/M
9. Blood Urea
10. S. Creatine
11. L.F.T.
12. Others

B. Semen Analysis

C Semen $\langle^C_S$

D. Special Tests
1. Hormones/FSH/LH/TSH/Testosteravel
2. Testicular Ultrasound (Color Doppler)
3. Diagnostic TESA for Azoo
4. Karyotype for Azoo

E. Sperm DNA
1. Fragmentation

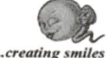

..........creating smiles

Fig. 2.42: Infertility test checklist

Parameter	SOH 1912
Volume (ml)	>2.0
Density (x 10^6/ml)	>20
Motility (%)	>50
Viability (%)	>75
Normal forms (%)	>30
Leucocytes (x 10^6/ml)	<1.0

Fig. 2.43: Sperminogram

Investigations

In case of abnormal seminal analysis we can follow the routine of investigation as given in **Figures 2.44 and 2.45**.

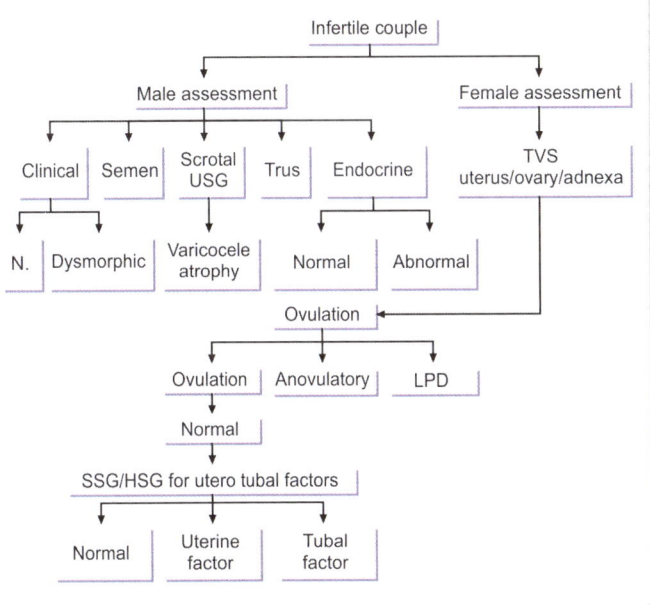

Fig. 2.44: Routine investigation of infertile couple

Workup of Female Partner

- History
- Physical examination
- TVS
- PCT
- Endometrial biopsy SSC/HSG (Tubal evaluation)
- Ovulation
- Assessment follicle

Basic tests		Special tests	
Male	Female	Male	Female
Semen analysis	TSH	DNA fragmentation	Endometrial receptivity assay (ERA)
HOS	PRL	Nuclear protein assay	Laproscopy
Vitality	Hormonal profile	Biomarker tests	Hysteroscopy
Morphology	HSG	Antisperm antibody test	APLA
Qualitative fructose		Leukocytes test	
Semen culture			

Fig. 2.45: Basic and special tests for infertile couple

- Monitoring
- Hormones (endocrine profile D2)
- Hysterescopy and laparoscopy

History

- Age
- Duration of marriage
- History of previous marriage with proven fertility
- Medical history esp. of tuberculosis, sexually transmitted disease, diabetes

- Surgical history especially of abdominal or pelvic surgery
- Menstrual history in detail
- Previous obstetric history
- Contraceptive practice especially of IUCD insertions
- Sexual history with problems such as dysparuenia, loss of libido

Examination

- General physical examination
- Reproductive system examination
- Distribution of hair
- Development of secondary sexual characters
- Per-speculum examination
- Per-vaginal examination of evidence of vaginal infection, cervical tear or infection, uterine size, mobility, abnormality presence of adnexal masses, and presence of modules in pouch of Douglas
- Physical features pertaining to endrocrinopathies.

Algorithms for Female Evaluation and Management

- Ovary
- Ovulation problems
- Ovulation induction
- Endometriosis
- Tubal factors
- Laproscopy

1. Ovary (Figs 2.46 to 2.48)

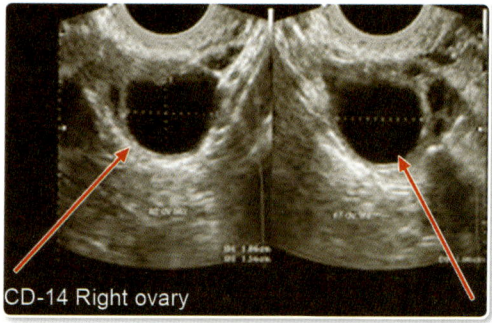

Fig. 2.46: Normal ovary

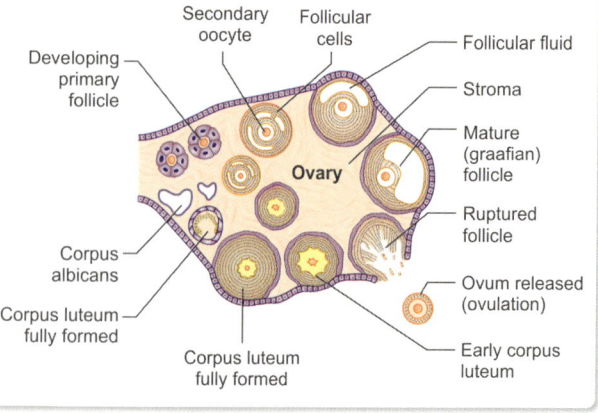

Fig. 2.47: Ovulation cycle

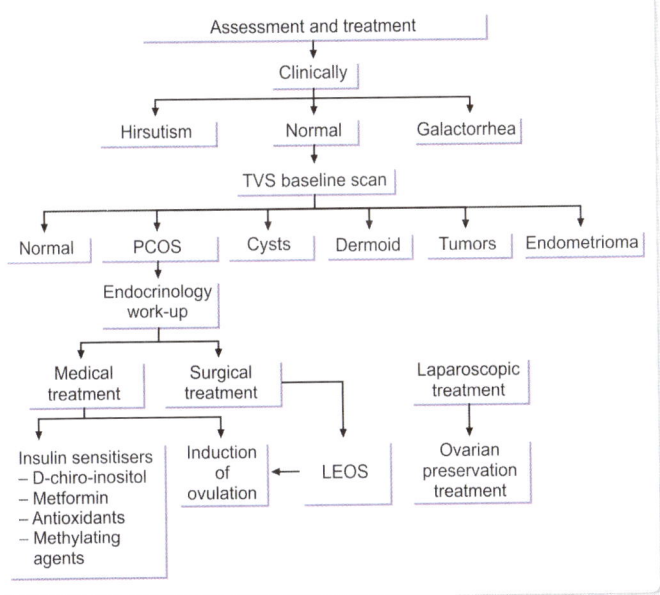

Fig. 2.48: Ovarian function assessment and treatment

Ovarian Problems (Figs 2.49 to 2.53)

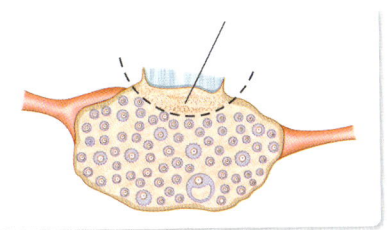

Fig. 2.49: Atrophic ovary

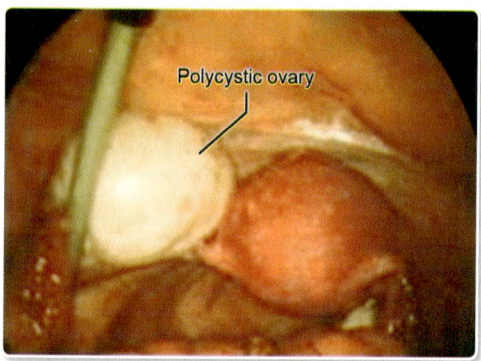

Fig. 2.50: PCOS ovary

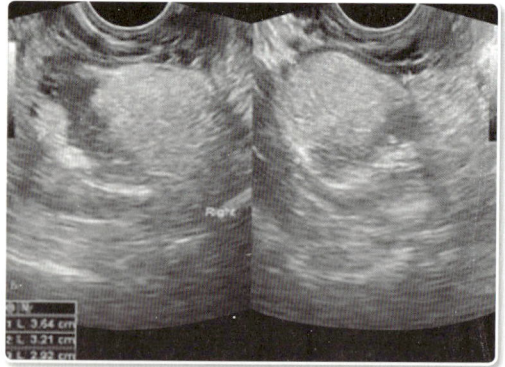

Fig. 2.51: Dermoid in ovary

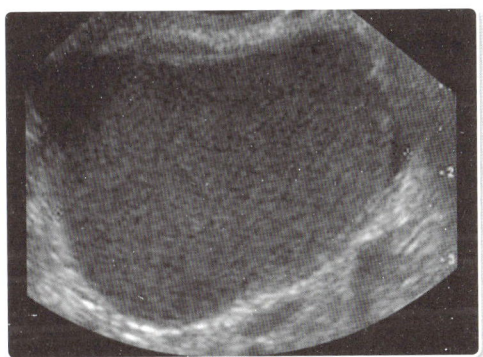

Fig. 2.52: Endometrioma

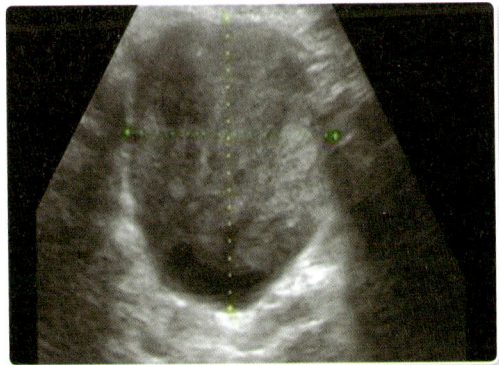

Fig. 2.53: Ovarian tumor

2. Ovulation Problem (Fig. 2.54)

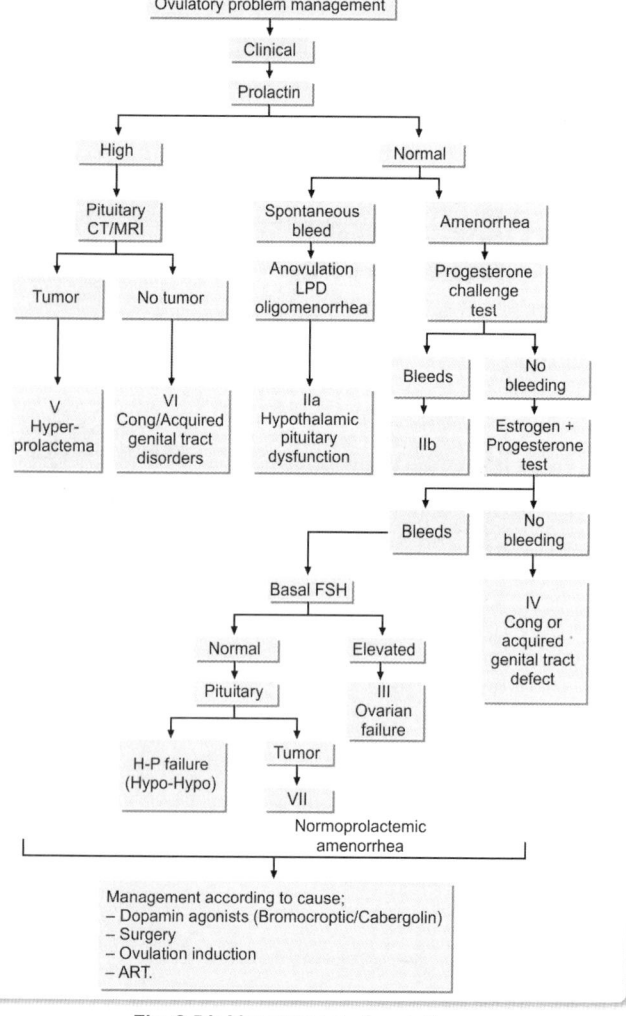

Fig. 2.54: Management of ovulation

3. Ovulation Induction (Fig. 2.55)

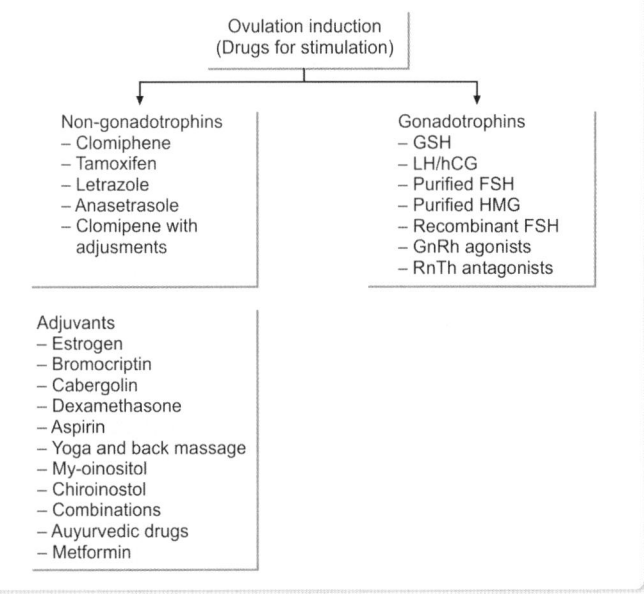

Fig. 2.55: Ovulation-stimulation agents

4. Endometriosis (Fig. 2.56)

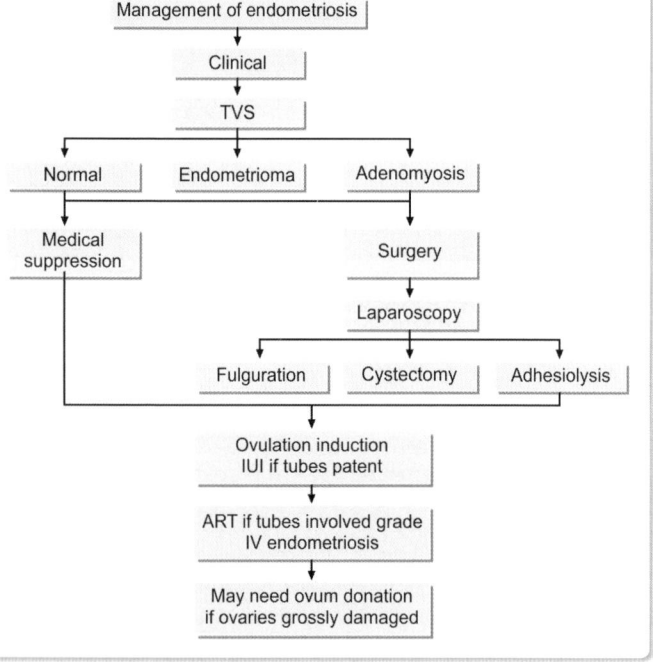

Fig. 2.56: Management of endometriosis

5. Tubal Factor (Fig. 2.57)

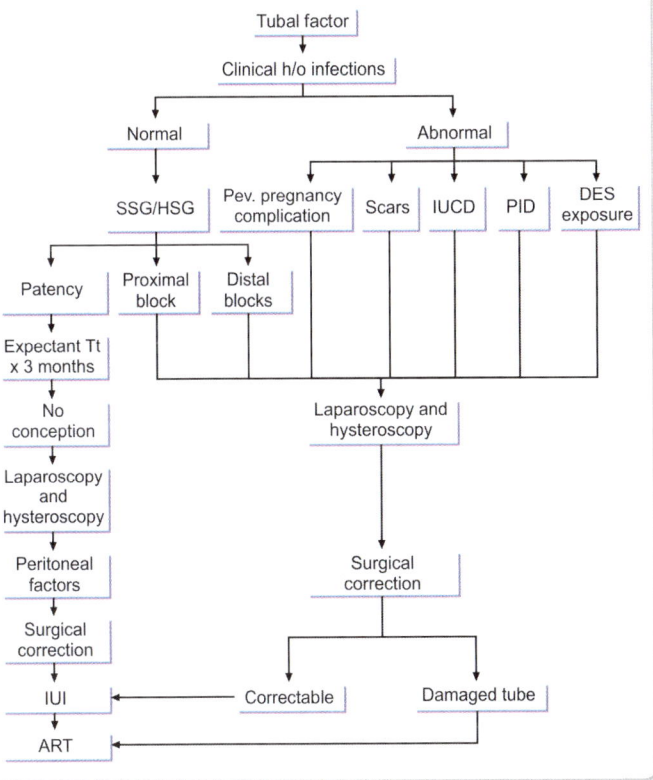

Fig. 2.57: Tubal factor of infertility management

6. Laparoscopy Algorithm (Fig. 2.58)

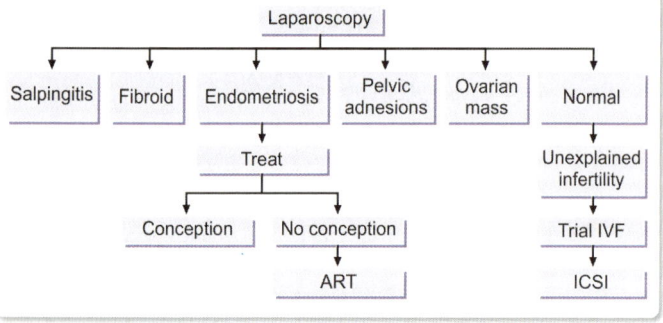

Fig. 2.58: Laparoscopic evaluation of infertility management

SONOSALPINGOGRAPHY STEPS

- Day 6–10 of menstrual cycle
- Sterile precautions
- Women on ultrasound couch legs folded (Lithotomy)
- Clean and Drape
- Scan TVS and document (uterus, ovaries, POD)
- Introduce SSG cannula/No. 8 french foleys/infant feeding tube
- Connect to 50 ml syringe with sterile solution (NS, Betadine, hydrotubation fluid)
- Focus on ovary, put color box on full screen
- Push fluid: see color bruit (Spill)
- Repeat on other side
- Deflate foley bulb, inject fluid to see cavity
- See pouch of Douglas for free fluid.

Luteal Phase (Fig. 2.59)

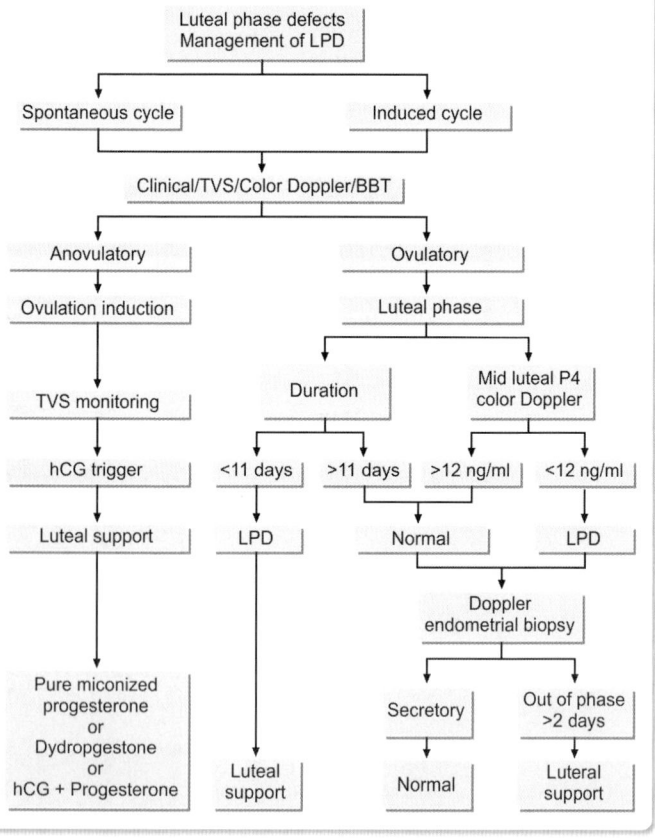

Fig. 2.59: Management of luteal phase defect

Work up of Male (Fig. 2.60)

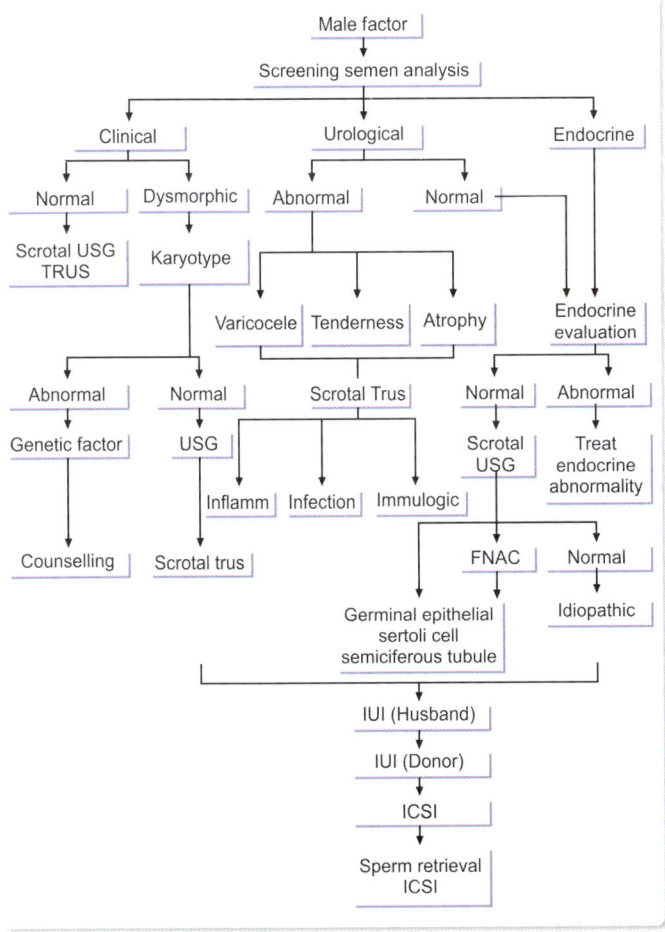

Fig. 2.60: Evaluation of male factor infertility

Abnormal Seminogram (Fig. 2.61)

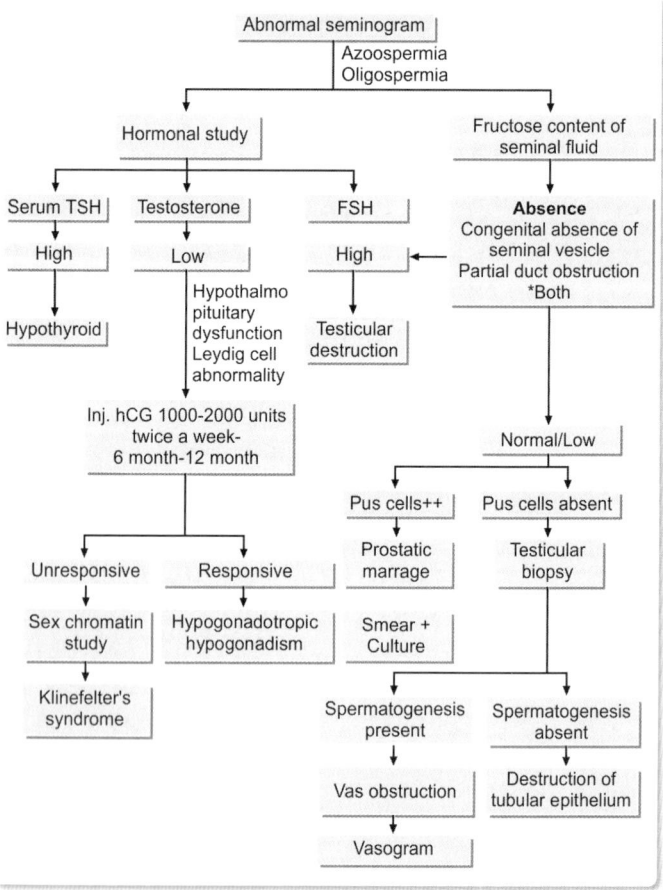

Fig. 2.61: Abnormal seminogram

Andrology Work Up and Set Up

Instruments and Accessories

Sperm Vision

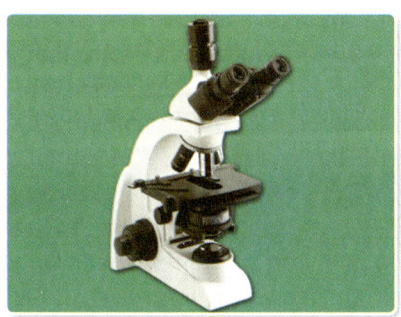

Fig. 2.62: Phase contrast microscope

In the laboratory andrology, routinely, there is a need of phase contrast microscope (preferably 10x and 20x phase optics with 40x and 100x bright field optics) with all standard configuration **(Fig. 2.62)**. Sperm vision is developed with following features.

Features
- UCIS infinity independent achromatic optical system.
- WF 10x plan eyepieces, 20 mm field of view, high eye point up to 21 mm.
- Seidentopf trinocular viewing head inclined at 300, Rotatable for 3600.
- + 5 diopter adjustment
- Phase contrast slides support for 10x and 20x objective lens.
- Quadruple nosepiece inward facing with positive click Stops
- –10x and –20x: positive phase contrast objective lens
- –40x (S): Plan achromatic objective lens

Practical Tips for Infertility Management

- −100x (S): Plan achromatic objective lens
- Rackless mechanical stage: 156 x 138 mm platform, with X/Y travel of 76x
- 54 mm by low-positioned X/Y coaxial control knob, with scale mark and specimen slide clip, enough space to hold 2 specimen-slide
- Coaxial coarse and fine focus mechanism with marking, fine focus sensitivity of 0.001 mm
- Centering telescope to adjust phase contrast
- Dust cover, clear blue filter, power cord, immersion oil.

Sperm Meter (Semen Analysis Chamber) **(Fig. 2.63)**

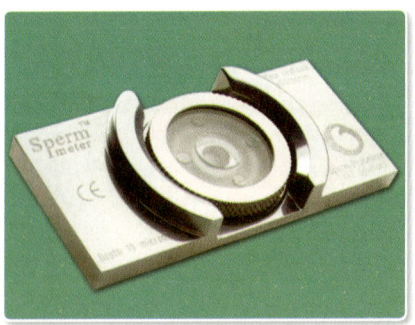

Fig. 2.63: Sperm meter

Preferably semen analysis is to be done without adding any diluents. Owing to viscous nature of semen, it forms a smear of distinct thickness. Hence during microscopic analysis dimensional consistency of smear thickness is an essential requirement, with this all the sperm should be in single layer avoids overlapping of sperms and free movement of sperm in all directions. Determination of precise sperm concentration and motility (Quantitative and Qualitative) requires well define micrometric area, preferably as surface graticule. The ultimate goal is Quantitative and Qualitative Assessment of sperm motility in terms of Sperm Concentration within the same focus of Microscope. 'Sperm Meter' Semen Analysis Chamber being design with following features:

Features
- Sperm meter has a metallic slide which can be directly mounted on microscopic stage without need for any accessories.
- Sperm meter has 10 μ depth optical window featured to bring all sperms in a single layer.
- Designed to eliminate need for semen dilution.
- Cover glass is with 1mm x 1mm surface graticules. Each graticule is divided into 100 squares each of 0.1mm x 0.1mm thus provides define micrometric area making it easy for calculations.
- Effect of air currents avoided.
- Enables to measure sperm concentration; qualitative and quantitative motility within the same focus of microscopic field.
- Design to use only 10x and 20x objective lens, avoid the use of 40x objective lens.

Sperm Warmer **(Fig. 2.64)**

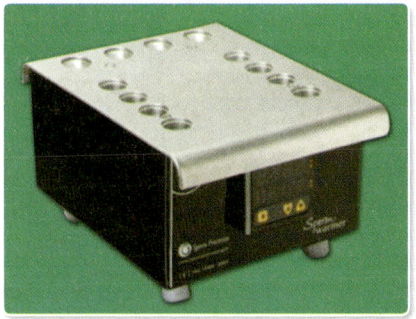

Fig. 2.64: Sperm warmer

The human body temperature is 37°C. Hence, ideally, the handling of the human gametes (sperm and ovum) during in vitro diagnosis should be exposed to 37°C ± 0.2°C so that the accuracy of the results in comparison to normal biological functionality is maintained.

The instrument has a provision to hold all the plastic ware, and disposable, such as semen collection containers, test tubes, vials, pasture pipettes, etc.

Features
- A single aluminum block containing heater and sensor programmed to attain and maintain 37°C ± 0.2°C
- Dual temperature system to display set temperature (Green color) and ongoing temperature (Red color).
- Accommodates sperm collection container, Test tubes, Angle tubes, Vials, Pasture pipettes, etc.
- Light weight.

Centrifuge Machine

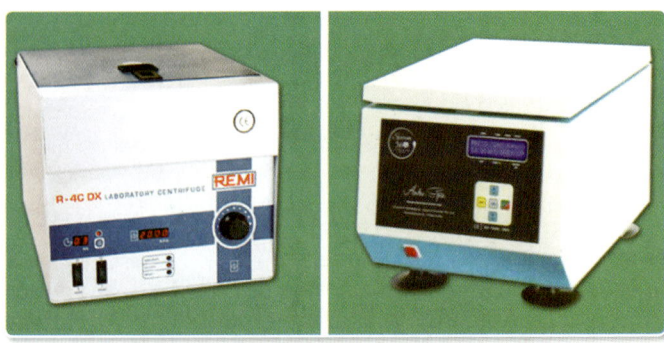

Fig. 2.65: Centrifuge machine

R&C Centrifuge Machine (CE Mark) with built in digital timer and step less knob to control the speed. Digital display of speed and image on screen **(Fig. 2.65)**.

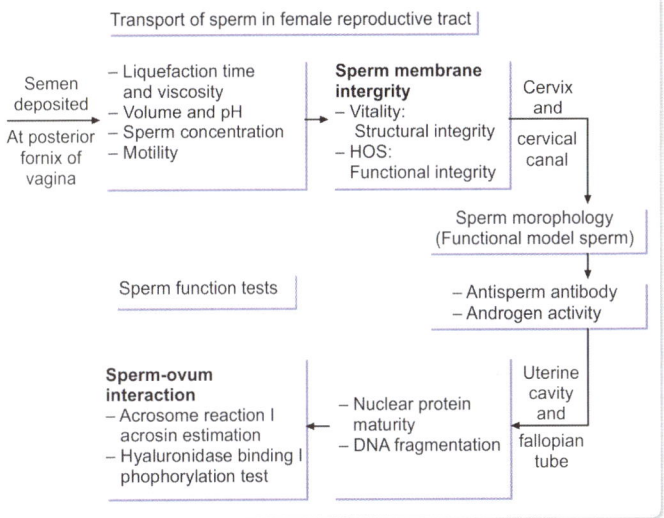

Fig. 2.66: Sperm transportation to uterine tube

Sperm journey in the reproduction track being is exposed to 37°C (Semen deposition, capacitation and fertilization). Hence during in vitro semen processing, if sperm is exposed to 37°C constantly, it helps to maintain its natural functionality **(Fig. 2.66)**.

To address the above said objective, Androspin has been designed to work at 37°C ± 0.2°C.

Main Features

- The centrifuge is programmed to set required RPM, time duration, acceleration, RCF, temperature in °C, Rotor no., etc for any given programmed no.
- The up and down button help to increase or decrease the numerical.
- The set temperature and current temperature are displayed.
- The automatic Lid lock is present.

Accessories and Disposables (**Fig. 2.67**)

- Slide staining
- DNA slide immersion
- Glass slide tray horizontal
- Glass slide tray vertical
- Volumetric pipette
- Micro tips box
- Glass slide stand (horizontal)
- Glass slide stand (vertical)
- Glass slide box
- Test tube stand
- Test tube holder
- Spirit lamp
- Kidney tray
- Coupling jar
- Scissor
- Wash bottle
- Marker pen
- Waste box
- **Disposable:**
  - Micro tips
  - Glass slide
  - Cover slip
  - Hand gloves
  - Tissue paper

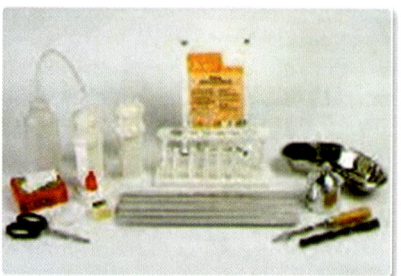

Fig. 2.67: Accessories used in andrology setup

Semen Examination and Processing

Liquefaction

- Take a sample from the laminar flow hood and record its details on your semen analysis sheet.
- Liquefaction should occur around 15–30 minutes post – ejaculate but if may take up to 1 hour at room temperature.

❏ Prolonged time to liquefaction (more than 2 hours) may indicate poor prostatic secretions since the prostate gland produces the majority of the liquefying enzymes.

Colour

A normal semen sample appears homogenous and opalescent. It may be less apaque if the concentration of sperm is low. It can also appear with a red or yellow tinge depending on the man's health and vitamin intake.

Volume

Measure the volume with the help of serological pipette. An average volume is between 2–6 ml per ejaculate. A very low volume may suggest congenital bilateral absence of vas deferens (CBAVD) since the seminal vesicles (which produce majority of a normal semen sample) are absent in this condition.

Viscosity

For checking out viscosity we do string test. Normal sample runs in small drops and viscous sample forms smaller or larger threads depending on its viscosity. High viscosity may interfere with analysis of motility, concentration, antibody coating.

String Test

❏ < 40 mm: Normal viscous
❏ 40–60 mm: Equivocal
❏ > 60 mm: Hyper viscous

pH (Fig. 2.68)

pH is measured with pH strip. Normal pH range for the semen is 7.0–9.0.

Measure the pH after volume and viscosity—by touching the "emptied" volumetric pipette to the test strip.

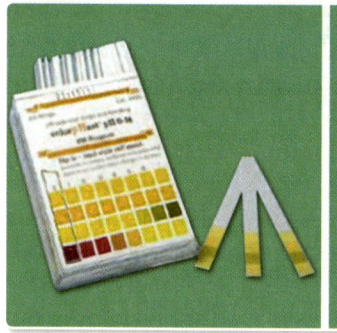 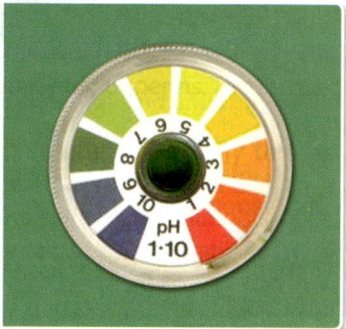

Fig. 2.68: Semen pH strip and measurement tool

Motility

- First make 2 smears to dry and use later. Prepare 2 frosted glass slides and label. Place 10 μl onto one slide and place the second slide on top and smear across both surfaces. Allow to air dry.
- Place 10 μl of semen on a clean slide and cover with a cover slip. Allow the sample to settle before viewing, before viewing, but do not allow the sample to dry out. A phase contrast microscope is best for this purpose.
- If >10% of the spermatozoa are involved in clumping, then the motility is assessed on the free spermatozoa and the agglutination is noted in the appropriate section of the form.
- Counting – select random fields and avoid selecting fields near the edges of the cover slips. Atleast 200 sperm should be counted and then percentage of motile cells calculated. You must distinguish between the criteria given in **Figure 2.69**.

R/L	Rapid and linear progression
NP	No progression but twitching
IM	Immotile

Fig. 2.69: Criteria of distinguishing sperm

- Sperm concentration _____ million/ml

- Sperm count _____ Million/ejaculate (Sperm Concentraton x Volume)
- Evaluation of sperm mobility:
  1.0 Progressive motility (PR)
      Spermatozoa moving actively, either linearly or in large circle, regardless of speed.
  2.0 Non-progressive motility (NP):
      All other patterns of motility with an absence of progression, e.g. swimming in small circles, the flagellar force hardly displacing the head, or when only a flagellar beat can be observed.
  3.0 Immotility (IM):
      No movement
- Total motile sperm _____ million/ejaculate
- Total motile sperm = $\dfrac{\text{Sperm count} \times \text{Motility\%}}{100}$
- Total non-motile sperm = $\dfrac{\text{Sperm count} \times \text{Non-motility\%}}{100}$

Agglutination: Agglutination is clumping of sperms into aggregates. Two types of agglutination occurs.

- **Non-specific agglutination:** Sperm cells adhere to various cell debris, leukocytes.
- **Specific agglutination:** Sperm cells adhere to each other in site specific manner like head to head, head to tail, tail to tail.

Site specific agglutination specifies immunological cause and anti-sperm antibody test conducted.

Select random field and avoid selecting fields near the edge of the cover slip. Score as given in **Figure 2.70**.

Rating	%
Not Significant	<10
+	10–30%
++	31–70%
+++	>70%

Fig. 2.70: Sperm agglutination score

Microscopic Examination of Semen

Parameters to be observed under the wet preparations
1. Sperm concentration
2. Motility assessments
3. Agglutination
4. Pus cells
5. Immature germ cells
6. Non-sperm elements

Bring all the sperm in single layer
Avoid the effect of air currents

Factors which affect:
- Choice of microscope
- Dilution of neat semen
- Depth of semen smear
- Air locking system
- Area covered for counting

Sperm Function Test

Semen Viscosity:
- **Kit Reagent:**
  Viscosity reagent – CH
- **Procedure:**
  - ***Step 1:*** Label plastic ware and disposable materials with appropriate patient ID and sample ID.
  - ***Step 2:*** Use freshly collected liquefied and well mixed semen to perform the 'String Tests', (Ideally use sample within 30–60 minutes after collection). Confirm hyper-viscosity of semen sample by performing the 'String Test'. Label the semen sample as hyper-viscous if the thread is of more than 4 cm in length.
  - ***Step 3:*** Measure the approximate volume of the semen.
  - ***Step 4:*** Add 10 µl/ml of viscosity reagent to the semen sample and mix well.

- **Step 5:** Keep well mixed sample at 37°C for about 10–15 minutes (maximum 30 minutes).
- ❑ **Examination:**
  Perform the string test at the end of the incubation and note the length of the 'string'. It should be 'Viscous' within normal limits.
- ❑ **Results' Interpretation:**
  Note the resultant viscosity.

Semen pH:
- ❑ **Kit Reagents:**
  pH Strips.
- ❑ **Procedure:**
  - **Step 1:** Label pH strips with appropriate patient ID and Sample ID.
  - **Step 2:** Lay the semen pH strip on a flat surface facing yellow circle upwards.
  - **Step 3:** Place a drop (about 10 µl) of liquefied semen on the yellow circle with the help of a pipette.
- ❑ **Examination:**
  Observe for the color change, after about 45–50 seconds of **step 3**, and compare it with the color chart printed on the strip.
- ❑ **Results' Interpretation:**
  The compared color match denotes the pH of the sample semen. Normal reference value/range: >7.2

Sperm Vitality
- ❑ **Kit Reagents:**
  Eosin-Nigrosin solution.
- ❑ **Procedure:**
  - **Step 1:** Label Plastic ware and Disposable materials with appropriate Patient ID and Sample ID.
  - **Step 2:** Take 50 µl of Eosin-Nigrosin dye solution liquefied semen.
    - Mix the dye and the sample

- ***Step 3 :*** After 30 seconds, place
- ***Step 4 :*** Allow the smear to air.

❏ **Examination:**
- Put a drop of oil immersion on the dry smear
- Examine the smear under the microscope with the help of 100
- Examine at least 200 sperm and count the followings :
  - Unstained/white sperm (Indicative of live sperm)
  - Red/dark pink sperm (Indicative of dead sperm)

❏ **Remark :** "Leaky necks", sperm stained only in neck region (heads remain unstained) are considered

❏ **Results' Interpretation:**
- Calculate the percentage of live sperm
- Normal reference value/range: 58% (55%).

Sperm Morphology

❏ **Kit Reagents:**
- Fixative solution
- Stain-I solution
- Stain-II solution

❏ **Procedure:**
- ***Step 1 :*** Label plastic ware and disposable material with appropriate patient ID and sample ID.
- ***Step 2 :*** Neat semen smear:
  - If Sperm concentration is greater than 20 millions/ml, place 5 µl of liquefied semen sample on glass slide. Form the smear.
  - If sperm Concentration is less than 20 millions/ml, place 10 µl of liquefied semen
  - Sample on glass slide. Form the smear.
- *Processed Semen Smear:*
  - Take a 100 µl of liquefied semen.
  - Add 200 µl of semen washing medium.

- Mix well, centrifuge at 2000 rpm for 2–3 minutes.
- Discard the supernatant.
- Use the pellet (5–10 µl) for preparation of the smear.
- **Step 3 :** Allow the smear to air dry
- **Step 4 :** Lay the smear horizontally and cover the entire smear with **1ml of Fixative** solution. Keep it for **15** seconds.
- **Step 5 :** Drain off the fixative solution and allow the smear to air-dry.
- **Step 6 :** Lay the smear horizontally and cover the entire smear with **1 ml** of **Stain-I** solution. Keep it for **10** seconds.
- **Step 7 :** Drain off the **Stain-I** solution
- **Step 8 :** Lay the smear horizontally and cover the entire smear with **1 ml** of **Stain-II** solution. Keep it for **15** seconds.
- **Step 9 :** Drain off the **Stain-II** solution
- **Step 10 :** Rinse the smear in DW
- **Step 11 :** Drain off DW and clean the back of the slide with a filter paper.
- **Step 12 :** Allow the smear to air-dry (use slide-warmer).

❑ **Examination:**
- Put a drop of oil immersion on the dry smear
- Examine the smear under the microscope with the help of 100X lens.
- Examine at least 200 sperm and count the followings as per Kruger's strict criteria/WHO criteria :
  - Normal sperm
  - Abnormal sperm
- In abnormal sperm, detailed abnormality (defects) pertaining to head, mid piece and tail should be noted down.

❏ **Results' Interpretation:**
- Calculate the percentage of normal and abnormal sperm
- Calculate total number of head, mid-piece and tail defects of the abnormal sperm.
- Calculate sperm deformity index and teratozoospermic index.
    - Sperm Deformity Index = Total No. Of Defects / No. Of Sperm Evaluated
    - Teratozoospermic Index = Total No. Of Defects / Total No. Of Abnormal Sperms
- Normal reference value/range : For Normal Sperm **4%** (3–4%)

Semen Fructose

❏ **Kit Reagents:**

Fructose Reagent : 1 x 50 ml

❏ **Procedure:**
- ***Step 1 :*** Label plastic ware and disposable materials with appropriate patient ID and sample ID.
- ***Step 2 :*** Take **1** ml of fructose reagent in a glass test tube.
- ***Step 3 :*** Add **0.1** ml of specimen.
- ***Step 4 :*** Boil it for **30–60** seconds.
- ***Step 5 :*** Observe the change of color.

❏ **Examination:**

Change in color from colorless to red tone to be observed.

❏ **Results' Interpretation:**
- If color changes from colorless to red tone, i.e. fructose is present.
- No color change fructose is absent.

Semen Processing

Swim-up Method (Fig. 2.71)

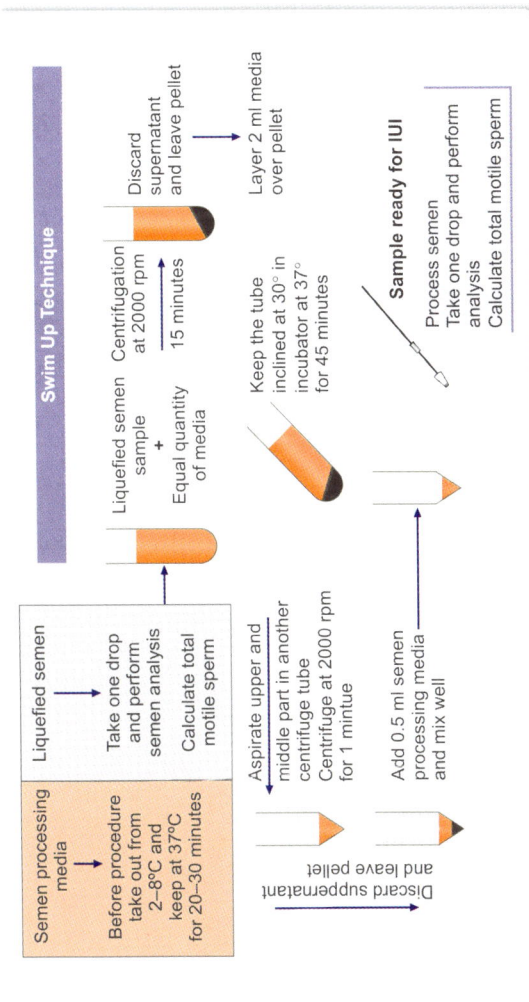

Fig. 2.71: Semen processing: Swim-up method

Density Gradient Method (Fig. 2.72)

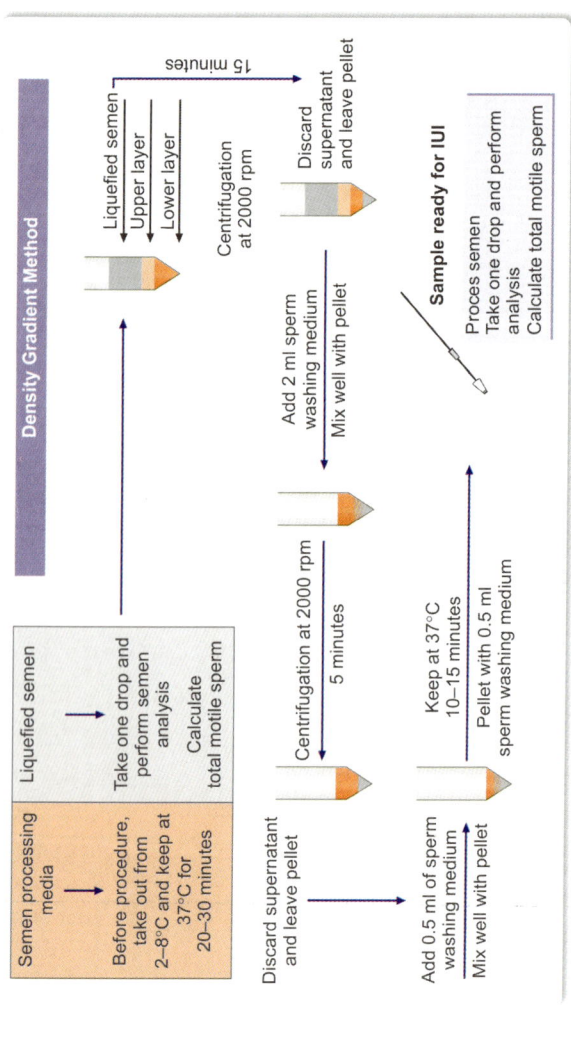

Fig. 2.72: Semen processing: Density gradient method

Assisted Conceptions

Infertility is defined as 'failure to conceive after regular unprotected sexual intercourse for 1 year in the absence of known reproductive pathology'.

Assisted conception treatments are often paired with fertility drugs to increase your chance of conceiving. The younger you are, the greater your chance of success of conceiving through these treatments.

For women under 35, the number of babies born as a result of fertility treatments is as high as one in three.

The various protocols used in assisted conception depending upon the investigations are as follows:

(a) IUI **(Figs 2.73 and 2.74)**

Indications IUI–Husband
- Female factors
    - Anatomic defects of vagina and cervix
    - Hostile cervical mucus/allergy to semen
    - Immunological factor
    - Sexual dysfunction (vagisnismus)
    - Mild to moderate endometriosis
- Male factors
    - Anatomic defect of penis
    - Sexual/ejaculatory dysfunction
    - Retrograde ejaculation
    - Excess or deficit semen volume
    - Semen liquification defects
    - Immunological factors
    - Male subfertility (oligo, asthenio or terato zoospermia)
- Others
    - Idiopathic poor post coital test
    - Combined infertility factors
    - Unexplained infertility

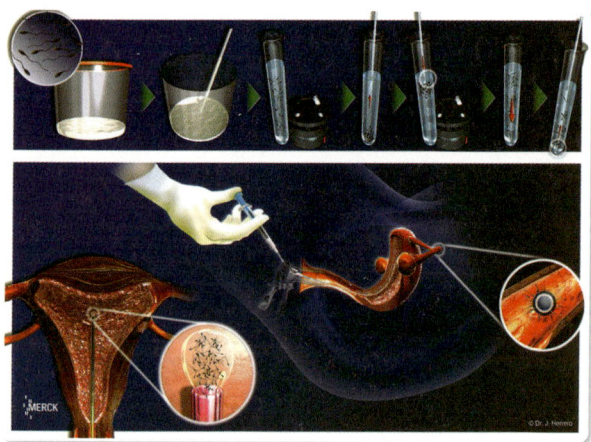

Fig. 2.73: Intrauterine insemination

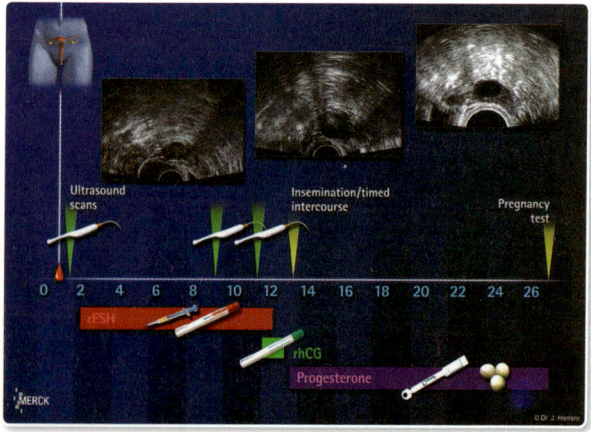

Fig. 2.74: Stimulation protocol for insemination/timed intercourse

Indications IUI–Donor
- Sterility due to disease, vasectomy, orchidectomy, chemical or radiation exposure

- Sexual/ejaculatory dysfunction
- Genetic disease
- Severe Rh incompatibility
- Non obstructive azoospermia/failed TESA
- Couples who cannot afford TESA–ICSI
- Single women and lesbians

IUI Procedure
- Ovarian stimulation
- Follicle and endometrial monitoring
- HCG trigger and timing of IUI
- Semen preparation
- IUI procedure
- Luteal phase support

(b) ART

- IVF
- ICSI
- Sperm retrieval techniques
- IMSI
- Time lapse embryo assessment
- Blastocyst

IVF
- Indications
    - Female factors:
        - Blocked tubes
        - Severe endometriosis (Grade 3 and 4)
        - Cervical factors
        - Anovulation (refractory)
        - PCOS
        - Failed IUI's
        - Immunological infertility
        - Long standing unexplained infertility

- Male factors
    - Oligo asthenospermia (Poor sperm quality)
    - Sexual/ejaculatory problems

ICSI

❑ Indications
  - Obstructive azoospermia
  - Non-motile sperms
  - Malformed sperms
  - Failed IVF-fertilization
  - Severe oligozospermia/globozospermia
  - Sertoli cell only syndrome
  - Rescue ICSI on 1 day old unfertilized oocytes
  - Antisperm antibodies
  - Ejaculatory disorders
  - Unable to give semen sample on day of IVF

Sperm Retrieval Techniques (Figs 2.75 to 2.77)

❑ Epididymal sperm (absence of vas/young syndrome)

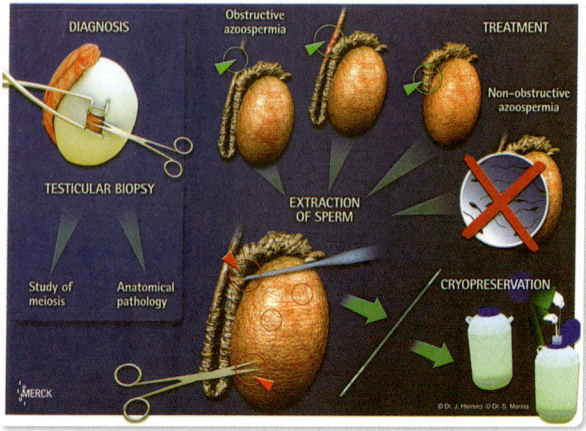

Fig. 2.75: Pathology of testes and seminal tract

An Approach to Infertility

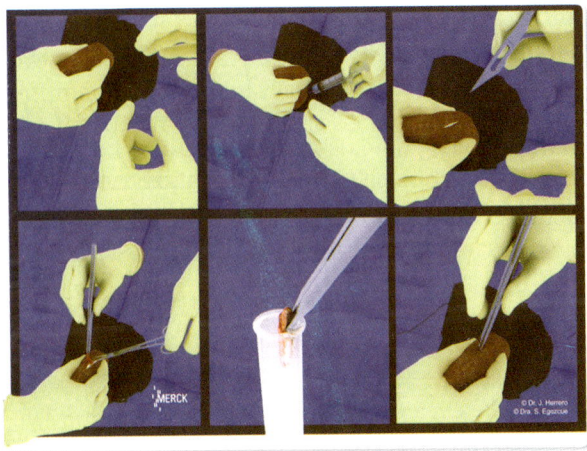

Fig. 2.76: Testicular biopsy

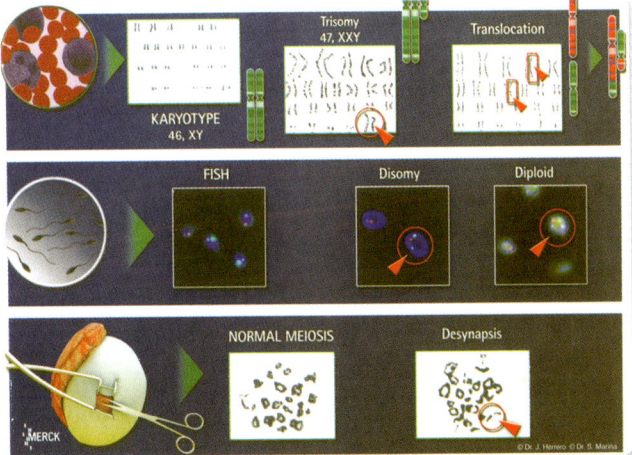

Fig. 2.77: Study of male chromosome

- ❑ Testicular sperm (focal spermatogenesis)
  a. MESA
  b. PESA
  c. SPAS
  d. RETA
  e. TESA/NAB
  f. TESE

IMSI

- ❑ Indications
  - Obstructive azoospermia
  - Non-motile sperms
  - Malformed sperms
  - Failed IVF-ICSI fertilization
  - Severe teratozoospermia
  - Poor embryo development in previous ICSI attempts
  - Good sperm selection morphologically
  - Patients with altered results in the study of sperm DNA fragmentation
  - Cases of long-term infertility with unknown origin

Time Lapse embryo Assesment

- ❑ Selecting the most competent embryo
- ❑ Kinetics of fertilization and early development of human embryos
- ❑ Kinetic markers of viability
- ❑ Timing and synchrony of cleavage stage of human embryos
- ❑ Significance of fertilization method and culture conditions
- ❑ Fragmentation and evenness of blastomeres

Procedure Steps of ART (IVF-ICSI-Sperm Retrieval)

- ❑ Patient selection
- ❑ Patient work-up

An Approach to Infertility

- Screening of both partners
- Down regulation
- Stimulation protocols **(Figs 2.78 to 2.81)**
- Oocyte recovery/ovum pickup.

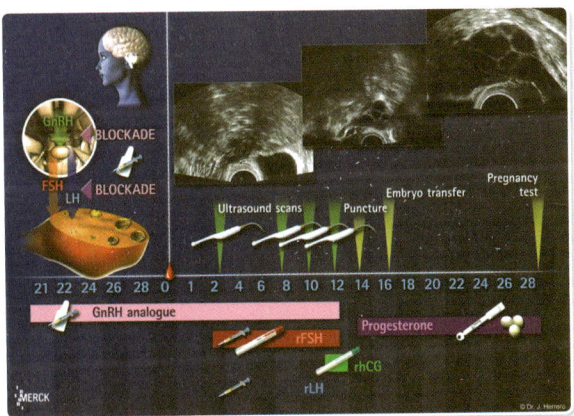

Fig. 2.78 : Ovarian stimulation, long protocol

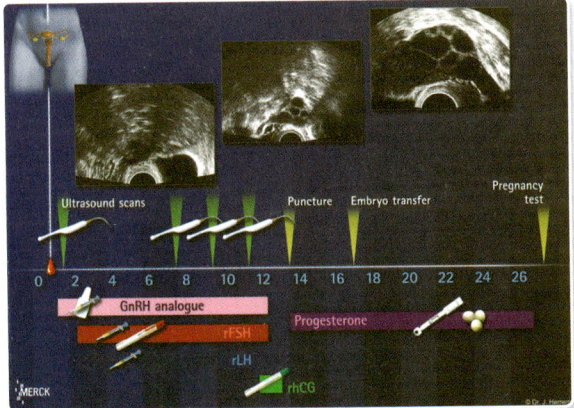

Fig. 2.79: Ovarian stimulation, short protocol

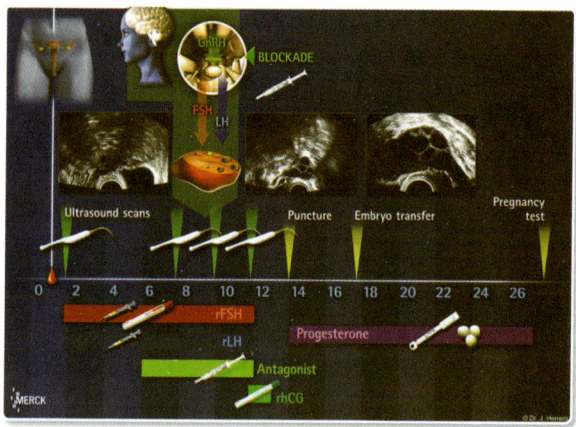

Fig. 2.80: Ovarian stimulation, antagonist protocol

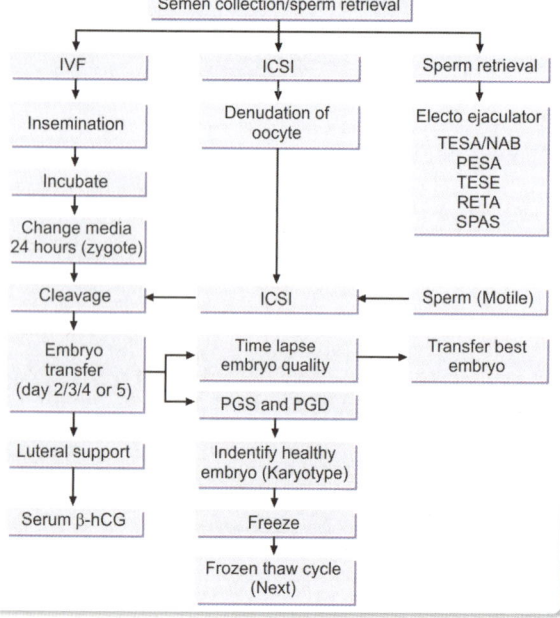

Fig. 2.81: Protocol of semen collection

IVF Steps (Figs 2.82 to 2.90)

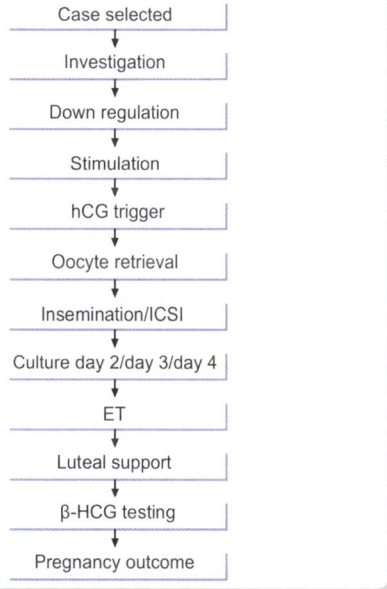

Fig. 2.82: Steps in IVF

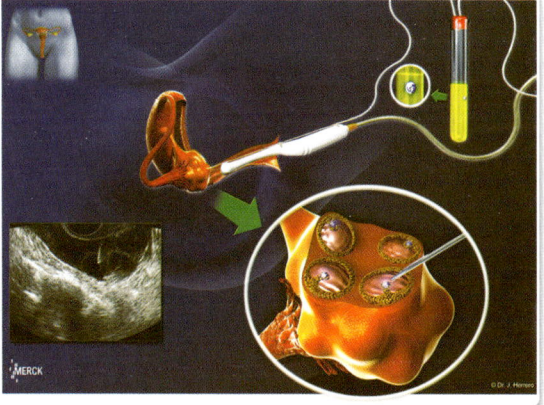

Fig. 2.83: Ovarian puncture

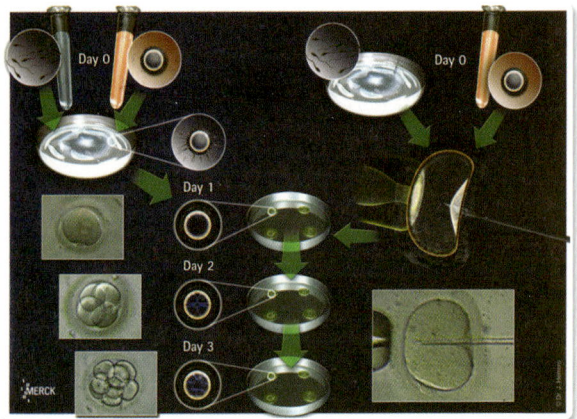

Fig. 2.84: The fertilization

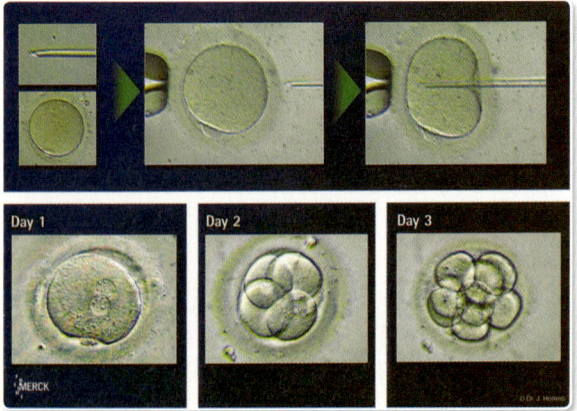

Fig. 2.85: ICSI fertilization and embryo development

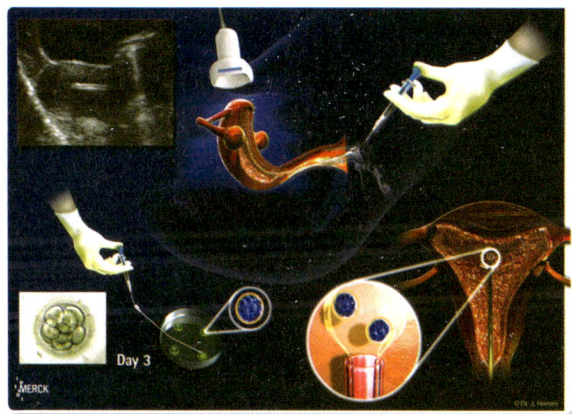

Fig. 2.86: Embryo transfer

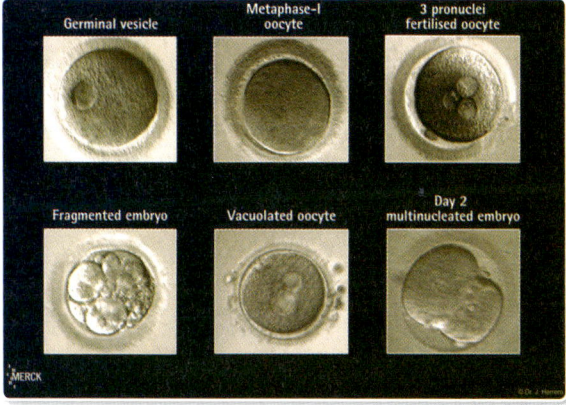

Fig. 2.87: Examples of oocytes and embryos

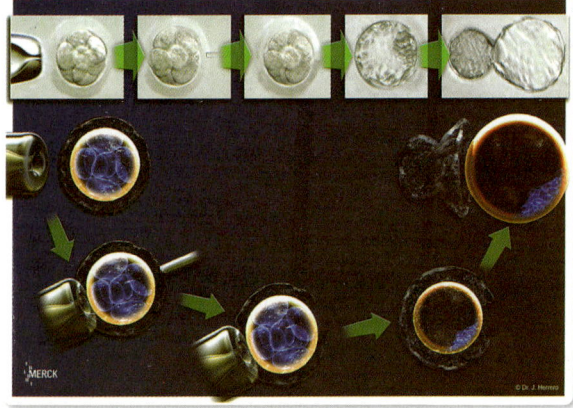

Fig. 2.88: Assisted hatching

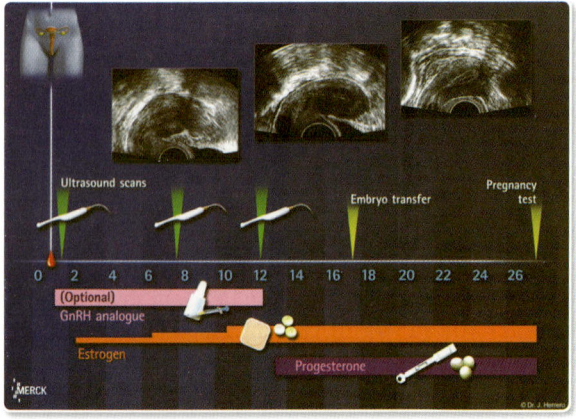

Fig. 2.89: Stimulation protocol for embryo transfer

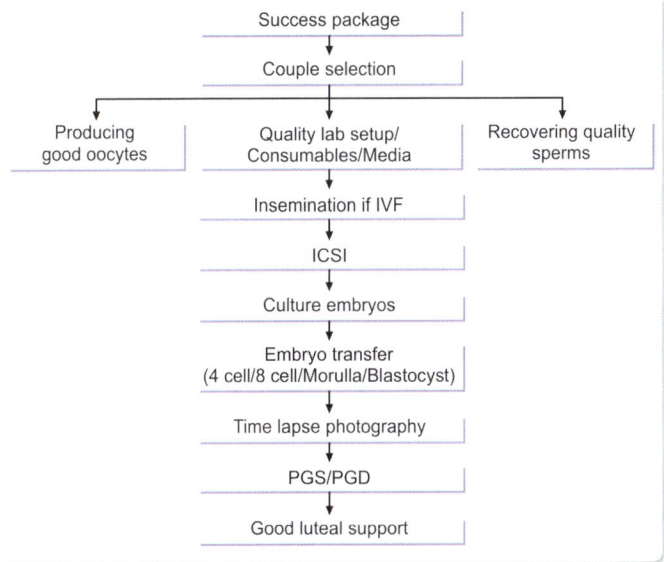

Fig. 2.90: Success package

Newer Advances

PGS and PGD

PGD and PGS are terms used to describe testing an embryo for a specific genetic disease it is at risk of inheriting from the parents. PGD is generally the diagnosis of a single gene defect in the embryo for couples that have a single gene mutation and want to ensure that their offspring won't carry the disease. Generally this group of patients has a 25–50% risk of transmitting a significant medical illness to their child.

PGS generally refers to the screening of chromosomes for aneuploidy (an abnormal number of chromosomes). PGS is the term used more often by reproductive endocrinologists when discussing infertility with couples struggling with issues involving age, repeated in vitro fertilization (IVF) failures, recurring miscarriages, or having had pregnancies that were genetically abnormal.

In patients carrying disease-causing single gene mutations, we recommend also testing for both the single gene defects as well as aneuploidy because we can do both at the same time. Some of the single gene disorders indentified using PGD include:

- Cystic fibrosis
- Hemophilia
- Huntington's disease
- Marfan's disease
- Muscular distrophy
- Thalassemia
- Tay sachs
- Spinal muscular atrophy
- Sickle cell anemia

On the other hand, PGS identifies embryos containing chromosomal abnormalities that result in IVF failure, miscarriage or babies born with Down's syndrome (Trisomy 21) or Edward's syndrome (Trisomy 18). Both PGS and PGD involve testing cells from embryo **(Fig. 2.91)**.

Embryoscope Time Lapse

Embryoscope time-lapse system is a unique platform facilitating improved IVF treatment, flexible work routines and effective communication, through comprehensive documentation of embryo development and evolving improvements in selection.

EmbryoScope® time-lapse system allows the uninterrupted culture of embryos whilst maximizing the amount of embryo development information collected. Evolving selection criteria

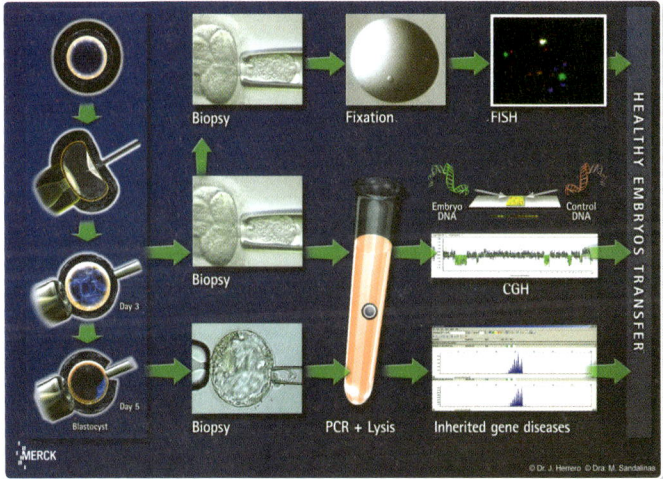

Fig. 2.91: Preimplantation diagnosis

are helping clinics worldwide to improve their IVF practise. Our solution constitutes a platform which is the basis for Improved IVF treatment and clinic digitization. EmbryoScope® time-lapse incubator offers:

- Undisturbed Stable Incubation
  - Tri-gas incubator allows fast and accurate regulation of CO_2 and O_2 concentrations with minimal gas consumption
  - Unique temperature control by direct heat transfer to individual media-filled wells. Temperature is virtually unchanged by opening chamber (<0.2°C) when adding or removing patient samples
  - Recovery of CO_2 concentration in less than 5 minutes and O_2 in less than 15 minutes after closing chamber
  - Continuous circulation and purification of air supply with residence time of less than 20 minutes

- Air purified by active carbon and HEPA filter. Removes VOCs and retains 99.97 % of particles larger than 0.3 μm
- Simplifies compliance with EU Directive 2004/23/EC by automatic logging of running conditions such as temperature, CO_2 and O_2 concentration to patient data files
- Dry incubation without water pans eliminates problems with water condensation and fungal growth on surfaces in high humidity

❏ Time-lapse Monitoring **(Fig. 2.92)**
- Fully automated detection and focusing of up to 72 embryos (6 patient culture dishes with 12 embryos in each dish)
- Image acquisition in multiple focal planes of all embryos
- High-quality Hoffman modulation contrast optics allows observation of key morphological features. Special Leica optics designed for red light at 635 nm to eliminate high energy light exposure.

Injection of G-CSF

G-CSF can help women improve endometrial thickness, according to new study from Center for Human Reproduction.

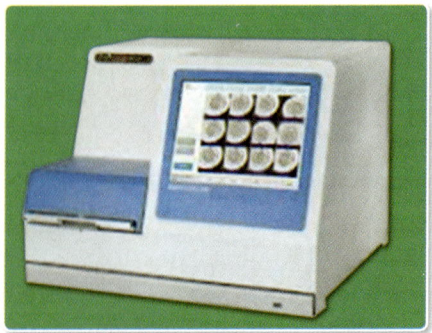

Fig. 2.92: Time lapse embryoscope

G-CSF(neupogen) is a cell-signaling protein molecule that can assist with maintaining the immune system in a "resting" state so it will not attack the embryo, it may increases the number of good quality eggs during an IVF cycle, increase the number of uterine natural killer cells (which assist in embryo attachment), increase embryo cell division, endometrial cell division and may even reduce inlammatory cytokine production. Patients with recurrent pregnancy loss that have been treated with G-CSF have shown higher pregnancy rates with no evidence to date of complications to mother or baby. Recurrent miscarriages that have failed IVIG, LIT and meet immunologic criteria for treatment.

Testing for Implantation Window

The endometrium is the inner lining of the uterus where the implantation of the blastocyst (an embryo that has developed for 5–6 days after fertilization) takes place. This layer experiences morphological and functional changes closely associated with the cyclical release of sexual hormones.

The term 'endometrial' relates to the endometrium. The ERA test works by analyzing the endometrial receptivity to implantation.

The endometrial receptivity array (ERA) test is a genetic test, which tells your doctor the best time for embryo transfer that would result into a successful implantation. It is a state-of-the-art diagnostic method, which was developed and patented by IVIOMICS after more than 10 years of research. This technique allows evaluating endometrial receptivity from a molecular point of view. This is done, by analyzing the expression levels of 238 genes related to it.

ERA test is conducted as follows (Fig. 2.93)
i. A routine endometrial biopsy is done in women undergoing their natural cycle or hormone replacement therapy (HRT) cycles, at a time recommended in the ERA literature (manual)

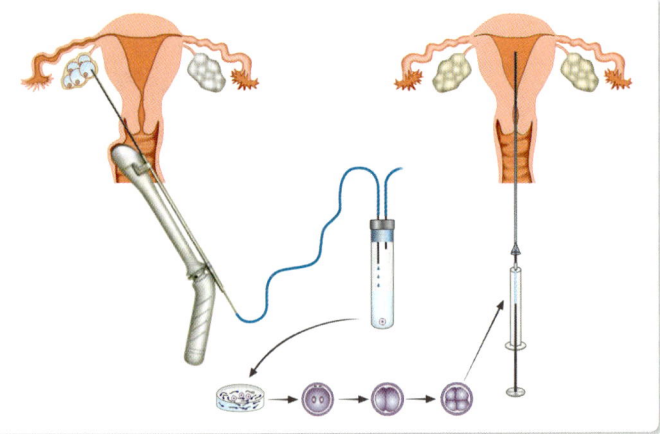

Fig. 2.93: Endometrial receptivity assay

ii. The biopsied tissue is then sent for processing and the results are delivered within 15 working days
iii. Based on the results, clinics can do the embryo transfers on the time suggested in the ERA report.

This test offers several advantages
1. It personalizes your fertility treatment by identifying the best time for embryo transfer
2. It reduces the chances of another emotional setback for patients.

Complications of Infertility Treatment

1. Ovarian hyperstimulation syndrome
2. Multiple pregnancy (high order)
3. Ectopic pregnancy
4. Depletion of ovarian reserve
5. Psychological disturbance due to failure

Ethics

ART guidelines have been issued by ICMR and forwarded to the Govt. of India for the formation of an ART act and to be incorporated with the PNDT Act of India.

Other Options

Options of third party reproduction like surrogacy still has no clear cut guidelines. Options of adoption should always be discussed with the infertile couple needing ART treatments.

Infertility Treated Pregnancies

- ❑ Precious pregnancies
- ❑ Close monitoring
- ❑ Slightly higher risk of pregnancy related complications
- ❑ Operative delivery in most of them.

Protocols for Freezing and Thawing

Semen Freezing

Swim-up

The advantage of this preparation technique is the high number of sperm with progressive motility and a very effective separation from bacteria and cell-debris. Swim-up can be used for normal semen sample. For semen samples with normal sperm concentration (>20 million/ml) but asthenozoospermia (40–50% motile) and or with teratozoospermia (8–14% normal morphology). Two methods are used:

- ❑ Swim up from pellet
- ❑ Swim up from ejaculate

Swim up from pellet procedure

It is the most used technique for separation of motile sperms and cellular debris. It is used with normal semen samples and is based on principle of active self-migration **(Fig. 2.94)**.

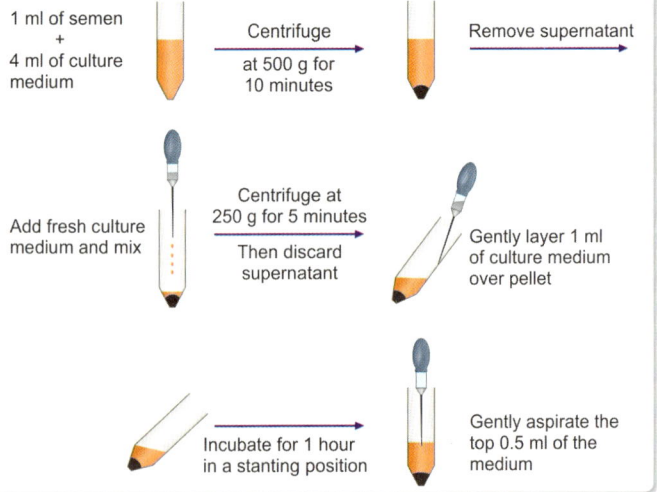

Fig. 2.94: Swim up from pellet procedure

- Label the falcon tube with correct patient name or code
- Add 4 ml of culture medium (HTF) and add 1ml of semen sample to it and mix gently.
- Centrifuge it for 10 minutes at 500 g.
- Remove supernatant without disturbing the pellet and add fresh culture medium and mix it well (Avoid backflow of the medium into the falcon tube).
- Centrifuge it at 250 g for 5 minutes and discard the supernatant.
- Gently layer 1 ml of culture medium over the pellet and incubate it for 1 hour in a standing position.

- ❏ Now gently and slowly aspirate the top layer of the medium around 0.3 ml.
- ❏ To this add 0.2 ml of cryoprotectent and freeze the sample in liquid nitrogen can by slow freezing.

Swim up from ejaculate (Direct swim up) procedure:

Also called Layering technique

- ❏ 0.5 ml of semen underlayed on culture media (HTF) as shown in **Figure 2.95**
- ❏ Incubate it for 30–40 minutes
- ❏ Pool out supernatant
- ❏ Spin at 1000 rpm for 6 minutes
- ❏ Discard the supernatant
- ❏ Resuspend the pellet with 0.5 ml of media
- ❏ Count the sperm and check the motility
- ❏ Freeze the sample for further use in IVF or for IUI.

Gradient Centrifugation

It is used mainly for the improvement of poor quality semen samples. It is used to fractionate human motile spermatozoa from other components of the ejaculate because of their

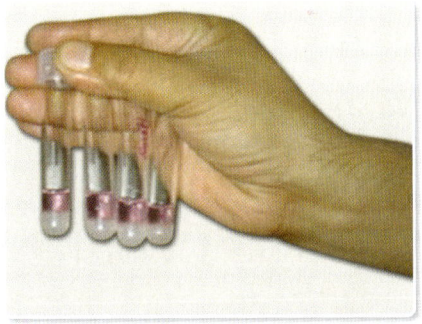

Fig. 2.95: Semen culture media (HTF)

specific density and motility. This technique is based on diff. in density and motility. It is the preferred method to select normal spermatozoa when there is more number of defective or dead spermatozoa.

Procedure

- Take one drop and put it on the makler chamber to take a count and determine the motility.
- Take two 15 ml conical tubes and label them with patient ID.
- 1 ml of 90% sperm gradient is layered in each conical tube with a sterile pipette.
- 1 ml of 45% sperm gradient is then gently layered on the top of it with another sterile pipette.
- 1–2 ml of sperm sample is then gently layered on the top of two layeres. Care is taken not to add too much sample as it result in poor separation.
- Without distrubing the layers, the tubes are centrifuged at 1500 rpm for 20 minutes.
- The supernatent is then pipetted out and discarded the leaving the pellet with as little of the 90% solution is possible.
- Take a new test tube and add 5–10 ml. Of flushing medium to it. Transfer the pellet to this tube **(Fig. 2.96)**.
- It is then centrifuged at 1500 rpm for 10 minutes. These supernatent is pipetted out and discarded. Add 5 ml media and repeat this step.
- And then placed it in to the incubator for 30 minutes. After 30 minutes, remove the 0.3 supernatent and put it in to the clean test tube.
- Add 0.2 ml of cryoprotectant to it and freeze the sample in liquid nitrogen can **(Fig. 2.97)**.

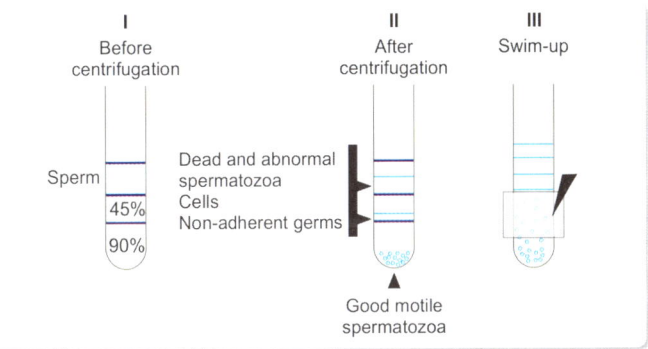

Fig. 2.96: Discontinuous density gradients (Percoll or alternative products)

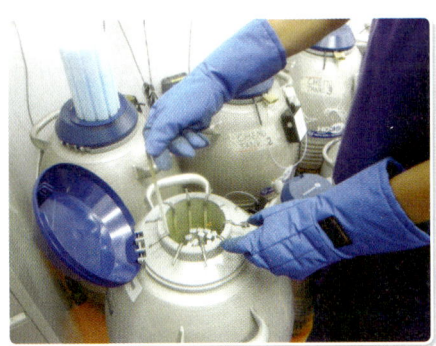

Fig. 2.97: Cryocans used for semen freezing

Embryo Freezing

Material Required (Fig. 2.98)
- Sterile petri dish (50 mm × 9 mm, Falcon 351007 or equivalent 4 well null dish).

- Transfer pipettes
- Disposable gloves
- Timer/stopwatch
- Liquid nitrogen reservoir
- Liquid nitrogen
- Cryotubes, Goblets, Cryocans

Reagents
- Equilibration solution
- Vitrification solution

Note: The warming and dilution procedure is to be performed at 35–37°C. Use a heated stage for the following procedures. Minimize the exposure of embryos to light during the procedure.

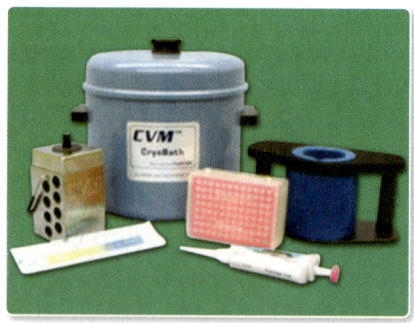

Fig. 2.98: Embryo freezing tools

Procedure

- Fill the liquid nitrogen reservoir with liquid nitrogen to a sufficient depth to submerge a cryotube or goblet on the cryocan and place near to microscope
- Determine the number of embryos to be determined.
- Label each sterile plate with necessary patient information.
- Make sure that the contents of each vial are properly mixed

- Prepare an inverted lid of a petri dish by aseptically dispensing one 20 µl drop of ES on the lid
- Remove the culture dish with embryos from the incubator and check the qualities of embryos. Whenever, possible use only the best quality expanded embryos for vitrification.
- Carefully transfer the embryos **(no more than two in one procedure)** with a minimal volume of culture medium to the drop of ES and start the timer. Allow the blastocyst to equilibrate in the medium for 5–15 minutes. The embryos will shrink and then gradually re-expand to its original size, indicating equilibration is complete.
- During the equilibration time in ES, set up 4 x 20 µL drops of VS
- After equilibration in ES is complete, draw up some ES into the pipette and transfer the embryos with minimal volume from ES to first drop of VS for 5 seconds.
- Quickly transfer the embryos to the second drop of VS for 5 seconds.
- Next, transfer the embryos to third drop of VS for 10 seconds.
- Finally, transfer the embryos to fourth drop of VS.
- Now pick-up the vitrified embryos in to the microtip and load it on loading device (cryo sleeve) **(Fig. 2.99)**.
- Quickly plunge this loading device in to liquid nitrogen.

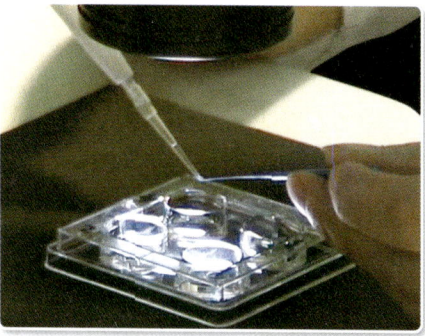

Fig. 2.99: Picking up vitrified embryo on microtip

Embryo Thawing

Materials Required
- Sterile petri dishes (50 mm × 9 mm, Falcon 351007 or equivalent 4 well null dish).
- Transfer pipettes
- Disposable gloves
- Timer/stopwatch
- Liquid nitrogen reservoir
- Liquid nitrogen
- Culture medium (culture dish)

Reagents
- 0.1 M sucrose warming solution (0.5 M WS)
- 1 M sucrose warming solution (1 M WS)
- MOPS solution (MS)

Note: The warming and dilution procedure is to be performed at 35–37°C. Use a heated stage for the following procedures. Minimize the exposure of embryos to light during the procedure.

Procedure

- Bring the solutions to 35–37°C.
- Fill the liquid nitrogen reservoir with liquid nitrogen to a sufficient depth to completely submerge cryo tube or goblet containing the carrier device used and place near to the liquid nitrogen freezer containing the vitrified samples to be warmed.
- Remove the goblets containing the samples quckly in to the reservoir containing liquid nitrogen.
- Place the reservoir on the laminar air flow near to the microscope. Label a sterile petri dish with necessary patient's information.
- Make sure all the contents of each vial (1 M WS, 0.5 M WS and MS) are well mixed before use.

- Prepare the petri dish by aseptically dispensing one 20 μl drop of 1 M WS and two drops of 20 μl of 0.5 M WS followed by three drops of MS of 20 μl.
- Now carefully open the cryosleeve and immerse the contents in to the drop of 1M WS. the embryos will float from the device in to the drop. Leave the embryos in this drop for 1 minute.
- Draw up some 0.5 M WS in to the transfer pipette and transfer the embryos to next drop of 0.5 M WS for 2 minutes.
- Then transfer the embryos to the second drop of 0.5 M WS for 2 minutes.

Note: the embryos will remain shrunken during exposure to 0.5 M WS. During this time set up 3 drops of 0.5 M MS.

- Transfer the embryos to the first drop of MS for 3 minutes.
- Then transfer the embryos to the second drop of MS for 3 minutes.
- Transfer the embryos to the third drop of MS for 3 minutes.
- Finally, transfer the embryos to a dish pre-equilibrated appropriate culture medium and incubate in a CO_2 incubator **(Fig. 2.100)**

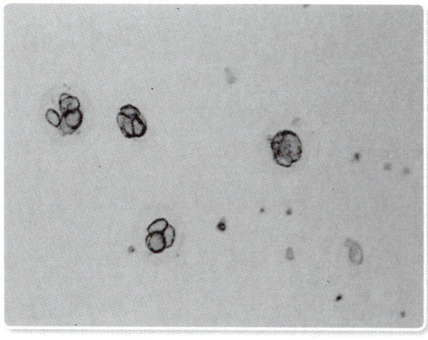

Fig. 2.100: Vitrified day 2 embryo in warming solution (0.5 M and 0.25 M)

Management of Infertile Couple (Figs 2.101 and 2.102)

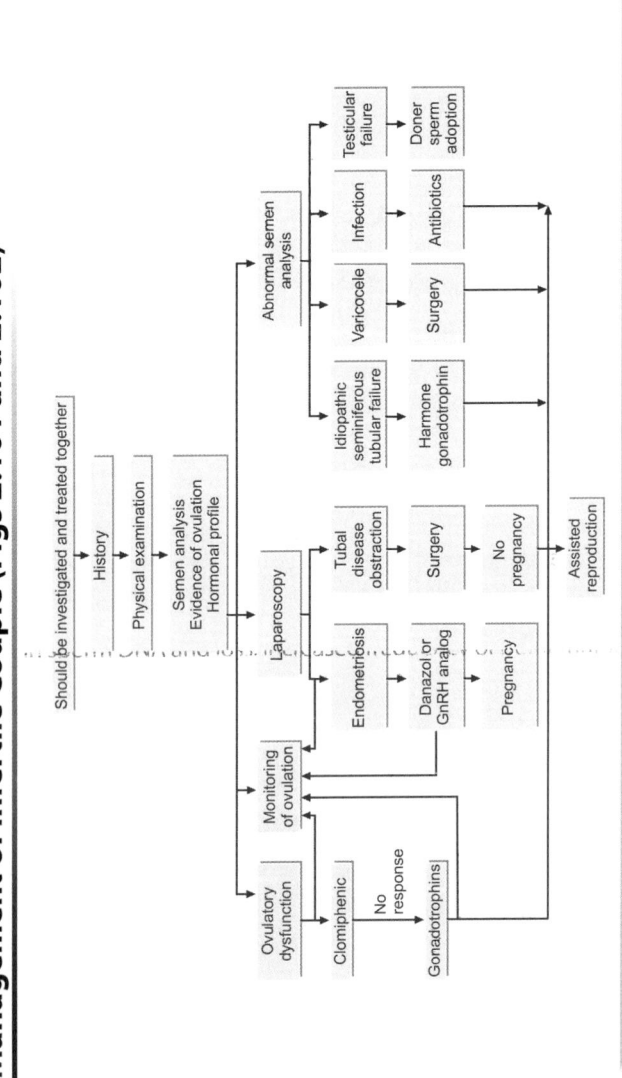

Fig. 2.101: Investigation and treatment decision

An Approach to Infertility

Identification of factor	Methods employed	Day of cycle	Observation
Ovulation	1. BBT	Throughout cycle	Biphasic
	2. Endometrial biopsy	21–23	Secretary endometrium
	3. Cervical mucus – Nature – Spinnbarkeit – Fern pattern	12–14 and 21–23	12–24 21–23 clear and watery Thick and viscid + — + —
	4. Vaginal cytology	12–14 and 21–23	12–14 21–23 Discrete cells Folded edges Pyknotic nuclei In clumps Background clear Background dirty
	5. Serum progesterone	8 and 21	8 21 <1 ng/ml >5 ng/ml
	6. Serial sonar	12–14	Follicular measurement 18–20 mm
	7. Laparoscopy	Secretory phase	Recent couples luteum
Tubal factor	1. Insufflation cycle	Proliferative phase-2 days after bleeding stops	1. Dropin pressure when raised to 120 mm Hg 2. Hissing sound in iliat fossa 3. Shoulder pain
	2. Hysterosalpingography	As above	Spillage of dye into the peritoneal cavity
	3. Laparoscopy	Secretory phase	1. Peritubal pathology 2. Pelvic pathology, e.g. endometriosis

Fig. 2.102: Contd...

Fig. 2.102: Contd...

Identification of factor	Methods employed	Day of cycle	Observation
			3. Evidence of ovulation
			4. Evidence of potency tube by dye test
Cervical	Post Coital Test	12–14	Presence of >20 sperm/high power field showing progression motility
Hormonal assay Done on day 2 of a spontaneous menstrual cycle	FSH (IU/1) LH (IU/1) E, (pg/ml) Testosterone (ng/ml) 0.24–0.89 (0.59)		**Normal Range/Mean** 1.6–6.1 (3.6) 2.0–10.5 (6.1) 44–53 (90)
Done on day 21 of a 28–30 day menstrual cycle	Prolactin (mIU/1) 150–500 Progesterone (ng/ml) >10		
	T3, T4, TSH B. Sugar – Fasting – Post prondial Evidence of sexually transmitted disease – VDRL – HIV evidence of tuberculosis – X-ray chest – IgA for active TB Sex chromatin study Evidence nuclerian – Buccal smear Evidence of pelvic inflammatory disease – Per-vaginum examination – Culture sensitivity of high vaginal swab		Thyroid abnormality Abnormal glucose tolerance test. Syphilis AIDS

Fig. 2.102: Identification and management of infertile couple

Protocols of Active Management (Figs 2.103 to 2.107)

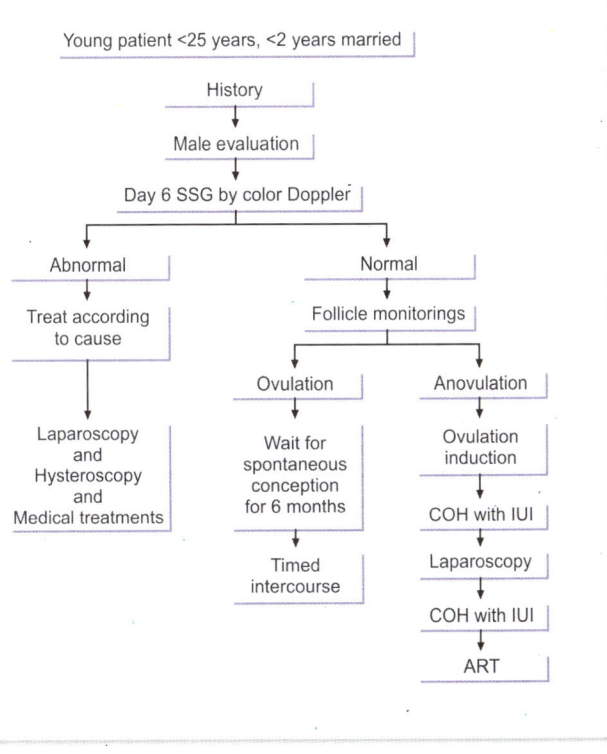

Fig. 2.103: Young patients <25 years, <2 years married

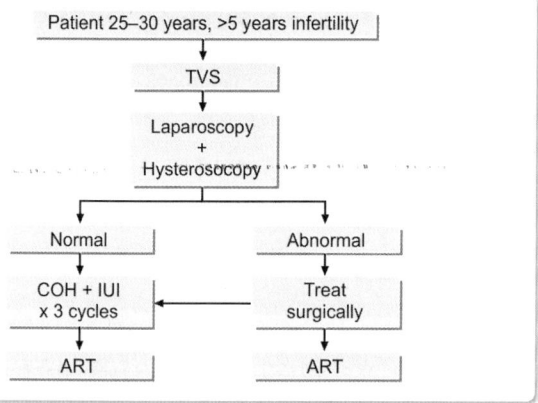

Fig. 2.104: Patient 25–30 years, ≥5 years infertility

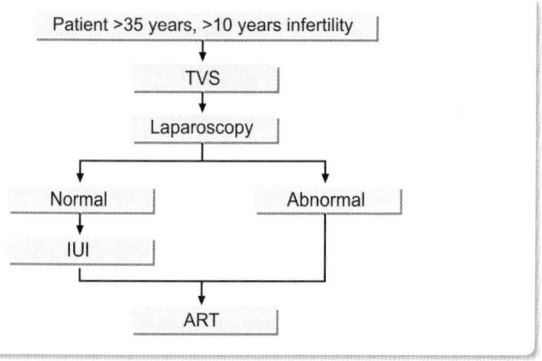

Fig. 2.105: Patient ≥35 years, ≥10 years infertility

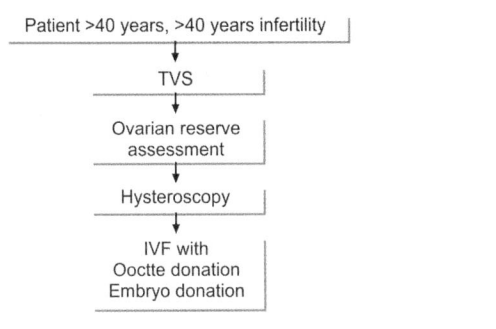

Fig. 2.106: Patient ≥40 years, ≥10 years infertility

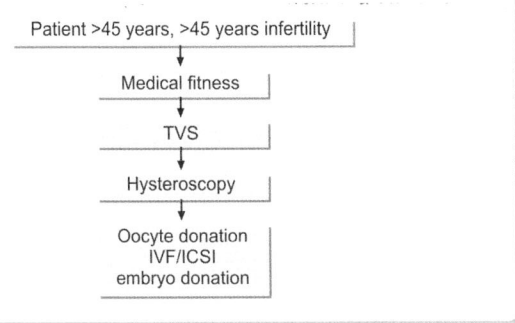

Fig. 2.107: Patient ≥45 years, ≥15 years infertilite

Infertility: FAQs

Chapter 3

Q1. Define 'Infertility'.
Ans. Failure to achieve a pregnancy after 12 months or more after regular unprotected sexual intercourse.
Primary—Never had a child.
Secondary—Failure to conceive following a previous pregnancy.

Q2. What is the male contribution percentage in infertility?
Ans. Males are the sole cause of infertility in approximately 20% of infertile couples and are an important contributing factor in another 20–40% of couples with reproductive failure (**Fig. 3.1**).

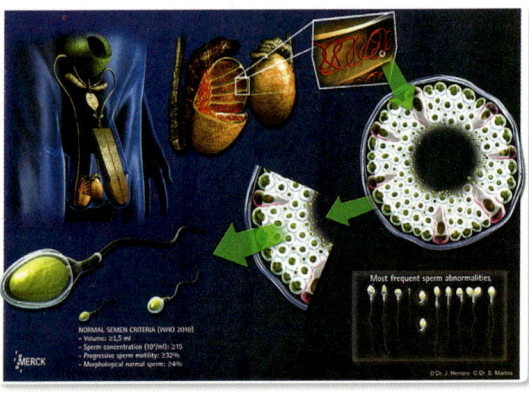

Fig. 3.1: Sperm anatomy: role in infertility

Q3. How long does spermatogenic process take to complete?
Ans. The spermatogenic process is directed by genes located on Y-chromosomes 4 and take approximately 70 days to complete. Another 12–21 days are required for the transfer of sperm from the testis to the ejaculatory ducts.

Q4. How do antisperm antibodies (ASA) affect fertility?

Ans. Approximately 10–12% men have ASA. Their presence may lead to a decrease in sperm motility and may impede sperm binding to the zone pellucida.

Q5. Does age affect male fertility?

Ans. Semen volume, sperm motility and the proportion of morphologically normal sperm but not the sperm concentration decreases gradually as age increases.

Q6. What is the initial evaluation of male factor infertility?

Ans. Initial evaluation should include detailed medical and reproductive history, physical examination and at least two properly performed semen analyses obtained at least 4 weeks apart.

Q7. Further evaluate oligospermia/azoospermia.

Ans. When a male presents with severe oligospermia or azoospermia, a hormonal profile of peripheral blood, including follicle-stimulating harmone (FSH), luteinizing harmone (LH), testosterone and estradiol levels, should be requested. In addition, in azoopermia, a karyotype should also be done **(Fig. 3.2)**.

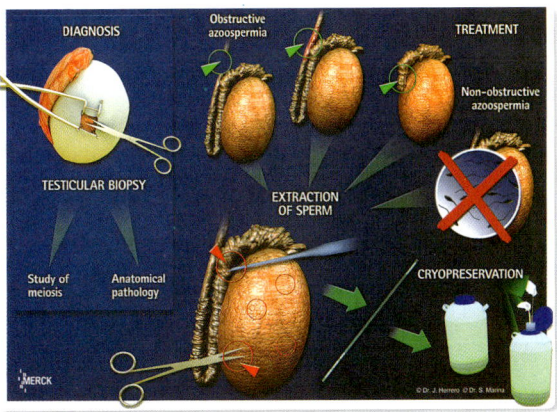

Fig. 3.2: Diagnostic evaluation and semen extraction

Q8. Does obesity contribute to infertility?

Ans. Obesity can lead to a condition known as metabolic syndrome (MS). MS causes infertility through:
- Excess adipose, tissue which causes conversion of testosterone to estrogen. Subsequently causing secondary hypogonadism.
- Increased scrotal temperature due to suprapubic and inner thigh fat.
- MS is associated with increased oxidative stress.

Q9. What is the effect of smoking?

Ans. Smoking leads to increase in reactive oxygen species (ROS) level and reactive nitrogen species, which causes low sperm count, decrease in motility and poor morphology.

Q10. Cell phones affect fertility adversely—Truth or Myth?

Ans. Microwaves produced by mobile significantly deplete superoxide dismutase activity and increase the concentration of malonyldialdehyde. This leads to decrease in sperm parameters.

Q11. What are the causes of congenital azoospermia?

Ans. Congenital causes include cystic fibrosis, congenital absence of vas deferens, ejaculatory duct or prostatic cyst and Young's syndrome.

Q12. What are the various sperm retrieval techniques?

Ans.
- Percutaneous epididymal sperm aspiration (PESA)
- Testicular sperm aspiration (TESA)
- Microsurgical epididymal sperm aspiration (MESA)
- Microsurgical testicular sperm extraction (Micro-TESE)
- Testicular sperm extraction (TESE).

Q13. What are the treatment options for varicocele?

Ans. Varicoceles are treated either by surgery (open with/without magnification and laparoscopy) or percutaneous embolization of internal spermatic vein.

Q14. How does maternal age affect fertility?

Ans. One of the most important factors that influences a couple's fertility is woman's age. This is because of a decline in oocyte quality.

Q15. Are contraceptives the culprits?

Ans.
- Yes, intrauterine device (IUD) users are twice at risk of infertility.
- Low monthly fecundity rates are noted in women who discontinued oral contraceptives.

Q16. What is ovarian reserve?

Ans. The resting follicle pool represents one ovarian reserve from which follicle will be recruited for maturation throughout life.

Q17. What test can identify the ovarian reserve?

Ans. Dynamic
- Clomiphene citrate challenge test
- GnRH agonist stimulation test (GAST)
- Exogenous FSH ovarian reserve test (EFORT).

Biochemical
- FSH, estradiol, inhibin B, antimullerian, hormone.

Sonographic
- Antral follicle count, ovarian volume.

Histologic
- Ovarian biopsy.

Q18. Which is the standard test to assess tubal patency?

Ans. Hysterosalpingogram (HSG), which is performed in the follicular phase. Besides being a diagnostic tool. HSG has been shown to be therapeutic as well **(Fig. 3.3)**. Approximately, 30% of patients, who have normal HSG, will conceive over the following 6 months.

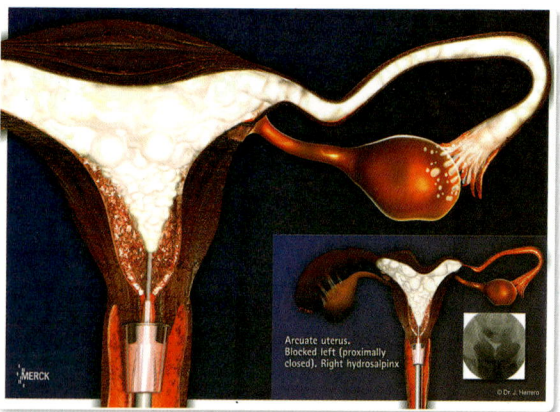

Fig. 3.3: Hysterosalpingogram showing arcuate uterus

Q19. When is laparoscopy indicated?

Ans. It is considered in patients who have a history of pelvic infection, signs or symptoms compatible with endometriosis or abnormal findings on HSG.

Q20. What is the epidemiological trend of natural fertility?

Ans. Natural fertility declines with maternal age. Normal women experience their peak fertility in early 20s and an accelerated decline in late 30s.

Q21. What is intrauterine insemination?

Ans. Intrauterine insemination (IUI) is a method of assisted conception in which washed spermatozoa are deposited in the uterus at any point above the internal os around the time of anticipated ovulation.

Q22. What is the advantage of IUI?

Ans. This procedure helps in overcoming the problems of vaginal acidity and cervical mucus hostility and allows deposition of a good number of highly motile and morphologically normal sperms in the uterus near the fundus.

Q23. What are the prerequisites for IUI?

Ans.
- Age <40 years.
- Patient capable of spontaneous/induced ovulation.
- At least one patent fallopian tube with good tubo-ovarian relationship.
- Sperm count >10 million/mL prewash or postwash >3–5 millon motile sperm with motility of >40%.
- Easy access to the uterine cavity via a negotiable cervical canal.

Q24. What is the regime of clomiphene citrate (CC)?

Ans. The drug is given in a dose of 50–150 mg/day for 5 days starting from 2nd to 5th day of the cycle. Starting from 2nd day reduces the antiestrogenic effect of the drug by the time ovulation occurs by day 14.

Q25. When is hCG administered?

Ans. Human chorionic ganadotropin (hCG) is administered when the leading follicle is 18–20 mm.

Q26. When to withhold hCG?

Ans.
- If there are more than 4 follicles >16 mm or >8 follicles >12 mm as, it can cause ovarian hyperstimulation syndrome (OHSS).
- If serum E2 >1500–2000 pg/mL.

Q27. How do we monitor follicular growth?

Ans.
- Transvaginal sonography (TVS)—Baseline on day 2, then from day 7 or 8 onwards.
- Serial serum estradiol levels.
- Urinary LH assay.

Q28. What should be the timing of insemination?

Ans. It should be as near to the ovulation as possible. 4 hours before or within 12 hours after ovulation yield good results **(Fig. 3.4)**.

Q29. What is the aim of ovulation induction?

Ans. Ovualtion induction aims to induce formation and ovulation of a single dominant follicle in an anovulatory woman.

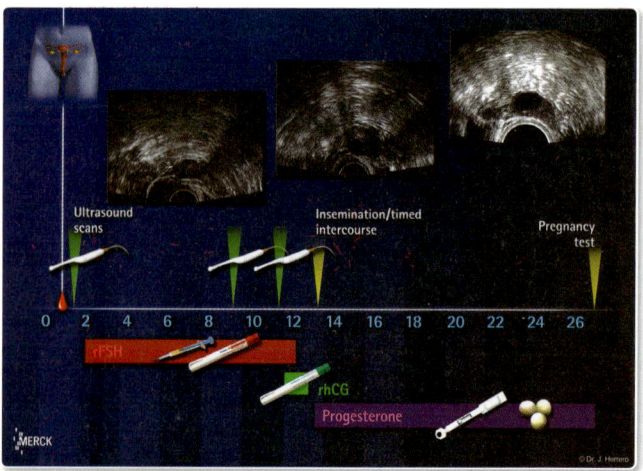

Fig. 3.4: Methods to know timing of insemination

Q30. Compare gonadotropin and CC for ovulation induction?

Ans. Gonadotropins are more effective than CC but are expensive, require parenteral administration and have higher risk for ovarian hyperstimulation and multiple pregnancies.

Q31. How does laparoscopic ovarian drilling help in improving ovulation in PCOS?

Ans. Electrosurgical reduction in the volume of ovarian stroma decreases ovarian androgen production and provides a better follicular environment. Reduction in androgen production causes lesser peripheral aromatization and elevated FSH levels and re-establishment of hypothalamic pituitary ovarian (HPO) axis.

Q32. What is the recommended procedure for ovarian drilling?

Ans. It has been recommended that a total of 4 punctures per ovary using a power setting of 30–40 W for a duration of 4–5 seconds per puncture produce an optimal response.

Q33. When to perform endometrial biopsy (EMB) in evaluation of female infertility?

Ans. EMB is not a part of initial work-up. It may be performed if the biphasic basal body temperature (BBT) curve is shorter than 11 days or if serum midluteal progesterone is less than 20, indicating a possible Luteal phase defect.

Q34. Which is the first test to evaluate uterotubal anomalies?

Ans. Hysterosalpingography.

Q35. When should an HSG be scheduled? Why?

Ans. The procedure should be scheduled in the midfollicular phase, which is 2–3 days after menses and before ovulation. It is scheduled after menses to decrease chances of retrograde flow of menstrual tissue and before ovulation to decrease the likelihood of women being pregnant.

Q36. Does HSG increase fertility by any way?

Ans. An HSG is thought to increase fertility by opening the tubes from the mechanical lavage of the dye, dislodging any mucous plugs and breaking down peritoneal adhesions. It may also stimulate the cilia within the lumen of the tubes.

Q37. Why is hysteroscopy performed?

Ans. It is performed to further evaluate abnormalities diagnosed by HSG or to surgically address these conditions.

Q38. Which women are at risk for diminished ovarian reserve?

Ans. It includes women older than 35 years, those who smoke, those with previous ovarian surgery and those with moderate to severe endometriosis.

Q39. What are the various autoimmune factors influencing conception naturally or by use of Assisted Reproductive Technology (ART)?

Ans.
- Antiphospholipid antibody syndrome
- Antithyroid antibodies
- Antinuclear antibodies
- Antisperm antibodies
- Antiovarian antibodies.

Q40. What are the major components of a woman's body for female reproduction?

Ans.
- Brain
- Ovary
- Fallopian tube
- Uterus.

Q41. What is the fertility rate of humans?

Ans. Overall, human beings are not very fertile with maximum pregnancy rates of only 20–25% per cycle during the years of peak fertility (second and third decades of life).

Q42. What cases should be exempted from 12 months' window period of inability to conceive as infertility?

Ans. Certain patients may have some recognized factors that would lead to problems in conceiving such as:
- Women with extremely irregular periods
- History of severe endometriosis
- History of previous tubal pregnancies
- Deranged anatomical factors
- Age >35 years.

Q43. Is infertility increasing?

Ans. Infertily rates are relatively stable but utilization of fertility services has increased because of the greater availability of services themselves and trend toward delayed child-bearing.

Q44. What are the basic tests for Infertility?

Ans.
- Transvaginal sonography
- Blood tests
- Fallopian tubes assessment
- Semen analysis.

Q45. What should we look for during a TVS?

Ans.
- Uterine abnormalities like fibroid/polyps
- Location of ovaries
- Antral follicle count (number of follicles present)
- Abnormal ovarian cysts such as:
    - Endometriosis, dermoid cyst, precancerous or cancerous lesions.

Q46. What blood tests should be performed?

Ans. Female—Blood type, blood count, rubella immunity, prolactin, TSH levels and hormone testing for ovarian reserve.

Q47. What factors determine ovarian reserve?

Ans. Ovarian reserve depends on two factors:
- Number of extra follicles available to undergo recruitment which depends on women's chronological age, previous ovarian surgery, genetics and exposure to environmental toxins.
- Actual health of follicles and egg within these follicles.

Q48. Should estrogen testing be performed with FSH levels?

Ans. Yes, because FSH levels can be misleadingly low in women, who have a high estrogen level early in the menstrual cycle.

Q49. Can a patient be normal with high FSH count?

Ans. Yes, she can be normal if TVS reveals a large number of follicles. With elevated FSH levels, she can be reassured about normal ovarian reserve.

Q50. How is clomiphene citrate challenge test (CCCT) performed?

Ans.
- In CCCT, a patient takes 100 mg of clomiphene citrate on cycle days 5–9
- FSH levels are checked on days 3 and 10.
- If levels are:
  - <10 IU/L → Normal response.
  - Normal on Day 3 and >10 IU/L on day 10 → Poor pregnancy rate.
  - >10 IU/L on Day 3 and <10 IU/L on day 10 → Borderline.

Q51. Does spillage of ejaculate out of the vagina after coitus affect pregnancy?

Ans. No, it is normal for much of the ejaculate to spill out of the vagina after coitus, and this does not decrease their chances of being pregnant.

Rarely, women with prolapsed vagina cannot support and hold enough ejaculate following coitus and can have problems with conception.

Q52. What is the relation between FSH levels and ovarian reserve.

Ans. FSH levels more than 15 IU/L are an evidence of diminished ovarian reserve. FSH levels exceeding 30 IU/L usually signify premature ovarian failure.

Q53. What is polycystic ovary syndrome (PCOS)?

Ans. PCOS is defined as the presence of at least two out of these three criteria:
- Irregular menstrual cycles
- Evidence of extra male hormones as determined either by clinical examination or by blood tests.
- Ultrasonography (USG), demonstrating ovaries with numerous small follicles (PCO-appearing ovaries).

Q54. Why should hydrosalphinx tube be repaired before IVF?

Ans. Women who have hydrosalphinx should have their fallopian tubes either removed or cut prior to undergoing IVF so that the tubal fluid, which would be toxic to the embryo or adversely affect the receptivity of the endometrial lining does not flow backward into the uterine cavity, preventing implantation of the embryo.

Q55. Does steroid use affect spermatogenesis?

Ans. One interesting cause of azoospermia is anabolic steroid abuse. High dose of steroids can supress sperm production. In such patients, sperm production can be reinitiated by stopping the steroids and placing men on gonadotropin therapy.

Q56. Which is the first-line drug for ovulation induction?

Ans. Clomiphene is the fertility drug of first choice for both ovulation induction and superovulation with IUI.

Q57. What are the precautions for males before planning IUI?

Ans. For men who have a low sperm count or motility, it is recommended that they abstain from sexual relations for 3–5 days prior to a planned IUI.

Q58. Do GnRH agonists have a role in IUI?

Ans. For most patients undergoing treatment with IUI, GnRH agonists are rarely necessary. These drugs are not routinely used unless a patient repeatedly experiences a premature LH surge during the treatment cycles.

Q59. Is IUI associated with some complications?

Ans. It is rare for any complication to occur after IUI. However, mild cramping or spotting can occur. Multiple pregnancy can occur in any situation when two or more mature follicles are present at the time of hCG.

Q60. How safe is multifetal selective reduction procedure?

Ans. This procedure is performed at approximately 10 weeks of pregnancy and involves injecting a salt solution into one or more of the gestational sacs. Overall pregnancy loss rate following this procedure is usually less than 5%.

Q61. Can ectopic pregnancy occur after in vitro fertilization (IVF)?

Ans. Ectopic pregnancy can occur within the section of the fallopian tube that passes through the muscle of uterus or within the short segment of fallopian tube. The incidence of ectopic pregnancy following IVF is 0.5–3%.

Q62. What is ICSI?

Ans. In intracytoplasmic sperm injection (ICSI), each egg is individually injected with a single sperm using tiny needle under microscopic guidance.

Q63. Who are the candidates for ICSI?

Ans. The common indication of ICSI is male factor infertility associated with an abnormal semen analysis. Another indication is unexplained Infertility.

Q64. What is sperm chromatin structure assay (SCSA)?

Ans. SCSA has been proposed as a means to predict the likelihood of pregnancy in cases of male factor infertility. This test analyzes the degree of DNA fragmentation present in a representative sample of sperm. Increased levels of DNA fragmentation seem to be associated with reduced pregnancy rates.

Q65. What is assisted hatching and how is it performed?

Ans. Assisted hatching involves weakening the zona to facilitate the emergence of the embryo following its transfer into the uterus after IVF.

It is almost always performed chemically. In this technique, a dilute acid solution is used to dissolve the external egg shell. Some clinics use mechanical hatching in which slit is made in the egg shell or even laser-assisted hatching.

Q66. What are the indications and risks of assisted hatching?

Ans. Most centers recommend this step in cases where female partner is >37 years, has dimished ovarian reserve with increased levels of FSH or is undergoing frozen embryo transfer with previously cryopreserved embryos.

There have been reports of increased rates of identical twinning following mechanical hatching. No evidence is there that assisted hatching harms embryo or causes birth defects.

Q67. What is ovarian hyperstimulation syndrome (OHSS)?

Ans. OHSS is a complication associated with the use of fertility drugs. Mild OHSS results in enlarged tender ovaries but only minimal fluid in the abdominal cavity. Moderate and severe forms of OHSS are associated with fluid accumulation in the abdominal cavity or sometimes in pleural cavity surrounding the lungs. In its severe form, OHSS can result in nausea, vomiting, shortness of breath and dehydration. Diminished blood flow to the kidneys may lead to diminished urine production. This situation can spiral downwards rapidly and complications of blood clot formation and kidney damage can occur if the patient is left untreated.

Q68. What can be done to prevent OHSS?

Ans. This syndrome can best be avoided by judicious use of fertility medications, and individually gonadotropin doses based on patient's history, the appearance of her ovaries on ultrasound and her previous response to fertility medication.

Q69. What is blastocyst transfer?

Ans. Patients who undergo an embryo transfer on day 5 or 6 after egg collection are referred to as having a blastocyst transfer.

If the embryos are maintained in culture beyond day 3, blastocyst forms on day 5. Many clinics maintain the embryos in culture until the 5th day to allow for improved selection of embryo to transfer.

Q70. What are PGD and PGS?

Ans. Preimplantation genetic diagnosis (PGD) and preimplantation genetic screening (PGS) are the techniques that provide diagnostic information concerning an embryo prior to its transfer to the uterus. The vast majority of PGD and PGS procedure are performed by removing 1 or 2 cells (or blastomeres) of a 6- to 8-cell embryo on day 3 of embryo culture following IVF. These cells are rapidly analyzed and on day 5, the unaffected embryos are selected for embryo transfer.

Q71. What is embryo freezing?

Ans. Good quality embryos in addition to those embryos that have been selected for embryo transfer can be cryopreserved by freezing them in liquid Nitrogen. The embryos are frozen at a temperature of −196°C, leaving them in a state of suspended animation in which they can remain for many years.

Q72. What are the pregnancy outcomes after thaw embryo transfer cycles?

Ans. The outcomes from using cryopreserved embryo has uniformly been positive with no increase in birth defects/developmental abnormalities.

In fact, many studies have shown that use of frozen embryos for transfer significantly improved clinical and ongoing pregnancy rates as compared to fresh embryo transfers.

Q73. When is embryo cryopreservation done?

Ans.
- It is done in cases where surplus good quality embyos have been left over after fresh embryo transfer in an ovarian stimutation IVF cycle.
- It is also done in cases who are hyper-responders with a risk of OHSS in ovarian stimulation cycles.

In these patients, fresh embryo transfer is withheld and all the embryos are kept frozen. Later on, when after the ovarian size decreases and estradiol levels drop, thawed embryos are transferred in a natural hormone replacement cycle.

Q74. What is egg donation cycle?

Ans. Ovum donation allows a woman to become pregnant when she is unable to successfully conceive using her ovum egg. In this program, donor eggs are obtained from healthy females of 21–35 years of age after stimulation of their ovaries with gonadotropins.

Q75. Who are the candidates for egg donation cycles?
Ans.
- Patients of advanced reproductive age-group, where the ovarian reserve and, hence, the oocyte quality, is already low. The number of eggs retrieved in such patients are too less for the patient to undergo any ART procedure.
- Patients with premature ovarian failure (age <40 years) are also candidates for egg donation. Premature ovarian failure may be idiopathic (70% cases) or iatrogenic as in previous ovarian surgery, chemotherapy or radiation therapy.
- Patients with known hereditary disorder like thalassemia, hemophilia or karyotypic abnormalities are also potential candidates for oocyte donation.

Q76. What is embryo donation cycle?
Ans. It is the transfer of an embryo resulting from gametes (spermatozoa and oocytes) that did not originate from the recipient and her partner.

Q77. Who are the candidates for embryo donation cycle?
Ans. Embryo donation cycle is an infertility treatment for those couples where both the partners have untreatable cause of infertility.

For example: A couple where the female partner has attained natural iatrogenic menopause and male partner is azoospermic.

Q78. What is gestational surrogacy?
Ans. It is an agreement where a woman (called a host/surrogate) carries a pregnancy with an agreement that she will give the

offspring to the intended parent(s). Gametes can originate from the intended parent(s) and/or a third party (or parties).

Q79. Which type of patients need a gestational surrogate?
Ans.
- Patients with congenital uterine abnormalities like absent uterus, hypoplastic/T-shaped uterus need a gestational surrogate to achieve parenthood.
- Patients with medical complications like uncontrolled diabetes, severe heart disease, renal disease, where pregnancy poses an increased risk to life of mother are also candidates of gestational surrogacy.
- Patients who have undergone previous hysterectomy due to obstetric reason like postpartum hemorrage or gynecological reason like carcinoma endometrium.

Q80. What does a cancelled cycle in Assisted Reproductive Technology (ART) mean?
Ans. It is an ART cycle (IVF/ ICSI) in which ovarian stimulation or monitoring has been carried out with the intention to treat but which did not proceed to follicular aspiration/egg harvested or in the case of a thawed embryo-to-embryo transfer.

Q81. What is ART?
Ans. It includes all treatments or procedures that include the in vitro handling of both human oocytes and sperms or of embryos for the purpose of establishing a pregnancy. This includes, but is not limited to, IVF and embryo transfer, gamete intrafallopian transfer (GIFT), zygote intrafallopian transfer (ZIFT), tubal embryo transfer, gamete and embryo cryopreservation, oocyte and embryo donation and gestational surrogacy.

ART does not include assisted insemination using sperm from either a woman partner or a sperm donor.

Q82. Is there a genetic basis for PCOS?

Ans. Yes, there is a strong genetic basis for PCOS, although the environmental factors can affect the degree and nature of symptoms. Paternal transmission of PCOS occurs 80% of the time when the father is affected with the gene. Maternal transmission occurs 45% of the time.

Q83. Is there any risk of acquiring viral disease like HIV/hepatitis during ART procedure?

Ans. No, as any other surgical procedure, ART procedures are performed under strict asepsis.

Q84. What are the chances of abortion after IVF? Are they increased as compared to spontaneous conception cycle?

Ans. The chances are the same as that of general population, around 15–30%.

Q85. Who are the candidates of IVF?

Ans. IVF is usually considered for the couples who have:
- Absent or blocked fallopian tubes
- Severe male factor infertility
- Advanced reproductive age as time to conception is critical and pregnancy rates with other therapies are low
- Other causes of infertility like-endometriosis, unexplained infertility
- Ovarian failure, although donor eggs would be required in this case
- When one or both the partners have inheritable diseases like hemoglobinopathies, cystic fibrosis which can he transmitted to the offsprings. In these cases, IVF with PGD is required.

Q86. Which kind of uterine fibroids needs to be removed before considering IVF?

Ans. Submucosal fibroids need to be removed by hysteroscopy before considering IVF. Also, the fibroids which are greaer than 4–5 cm size and intramutral should be operated upon before IVF as these tend to grow in pregnancy because of increased estrogen levels.

Q87. 'Advanced Reproductive Age' is a commonly used term in infertility patients. What does this really imply?

Ans. There is no universal definition of advanced reproductive age in women in part because the effects of increasing age occur as a continuum rather than as a threshold effect. Fertility clearly declines with advancing age, especially after the mid 30 seconds and women who conceive are at greater risk of pregnancy complications.

Q88. What is the effect of advanced paternal age on the reproductive outcomes in ART?

Ans. Increasing paternal age has been associated with more breaks in sperm DNA and loss, increased frequency of point mutation.

Semen volume, sperm molility and percentage of normal sperms decline with increasing paternal age. In turn, these are associated with increased time to pregnancy and decreased pregnancy rates. However, only a few studies have examined these outcomes adjusted for female age.

Q89. Can stress levels affect the outcome of ART?

Ans. There is an evidence in literature to suggest that stress levels influence the outcomes of infertility treatment as well as contribute to a patient's decision to continue treatment. Psychological distress is associated with treatment failure and interventions to relieve stress are associated with increased pregnancy rates.

Q90. What if the eggs do not fertilize in IVF cycle?

Ans. Most of the eggs will fertilize when they are placed in the culture dish with several thousand motile sperms. This is called in vitro fertilization.

In case the normal motile sperms, especially the fast progressive ones, are low in number, then the patient is taken up for ICSI cycle in which a single live sperm (after immobilization) is injected into each egg. On rare occasions, fertilization may not occur even with ICSI. This may be due to inherently defective sperms/eggs with a poor quality. In these cases, the use of donor sperms or donor egg may be required.

Q91. What are the success rates of ART?

Ans. Success rates vary with the age of patients, and also depend upon the infertility diagnosis and upon the experience of the clinic performing ART.

Success rates as per the age of the patients are given as follows:

Below (%)	Age (years)
40	<35
32	35–37
22	38–40
12	41–42
5	43–44
1	≥44

Q92. What is the most common complication of ART?

Ans. Multifetal pregnancy is the most common complication of ART. This can be prevented/minimized by limiting the number of embryos transferred to the uterus.

Q93. When does one get to know the outcome of IVF/ICSI cycle?

Ans. The patient is asked to get Serum β-hCG levels (in blood) after 14 days of embryo transfer.

Levels of β-hCG, if <2U/ml are considered to be the negative outcomes after ART cycle.

Q94. What are the rates of congenital malformation in the child born out of IVF/ICSI cycle?

Ans. They are the same as that in the general population, around ~3% IVF/ICSI cycle does not increase the risk of congenital malformations in children born out of ART.

Q95. In cases of male infertility, when is genetic testing required? What tests need to be done?

Ans. Tests for karyotyping and Y-chromosome microdilution need to be done when the male partner has severe oligozoospermia or azoospermia.

This is because these genetic abnormalities can be passed on to the children born after ICSI cycles.

Q96. What are the indications of hysteroscopy and laparoscopy while undergoing infertility treatment?

Ans. Hysteroscopy and laparoscopy are usually indicated in the following cases:
- When HSG (tubal patency test) shows evidence of blocked tubes or uterine cavity abnormalities like filling defects.
- Previous history of repeated failed IUI treatment.
- Ultrasound suggestive of abnormalities, such as fibroid uterus, endometriosis, hydrosalphinx, etc.

Q97. What is the first line treatment of infertility in PCOS patients?

Ans. Lifestyle modification and weight reduction are first line treatment of PCOS patients. It has been seen that even a 5–10% decrease in body weight in such patients is associated with improved ovulatory function. Weight reduction also improves the results of drugs used for inducing ovulation and decreases the doses of such drugs used. Also there is decreased rate of pregnancy complications like hypertension, diabetes, etc. when the patients have already lost weight prior to conception.

Q98. What is the link between infertility and endometriosis?

Ans. About 40% of women with infertility have endometriosis. Inflammation from endometriosis may damage sperm or egg, or interfere with their movement through the fallopian tube and uterus.

In severe grades of endometriosis, there may be adhesions/scarring around the fallopian tubes, which may cause tubal kinking/blockade.

Q99. Are there any chances of recurrence of endometriosis/endometrioma after surgical cure?

Ans. Around 40–80% (average 50%) of patients have recurrence of disease within 2 years after initial surgical cure.

There are no medications that can totally eliminate the disease. These drugs can only suppress the disease for some time.

Appendix

Table 1: Levels of hemoglobin

Level of hemoglobin	Health status
12 g/dl or above 12 g/dl	Normal
Below 12 g/dl	Anemic
10 g/dl–12 g/dl	Mildly anemic
8 g/dl–10 g/dl	Moderately anemic
Below 8 g/dl	Severly anemic

Table 2: Clinical and biochemical characteristics of the study population and mean hormonal values

	Entire group	Reference range
Total number	28	–
Age	55 ± 11	–
Male/female	4 ± 24	–
BMI	27.7 ± 4.9	19.5–24.5 kg/m^2
Glycemia	9.3 ± 18.5	70–110 mg/dL
Total cholesterol	200 ± 42	120–220 mg/dL
LDL cholesterol	129 ± 37	<160 mg/dL
HDL cholesterol	51 ± 15	35–80 mg/dL
Triglycerides	124 ± 43	50–180 mg/dL
fT3	2.49 ± 0.65	2.5–3.9 pg/mL
fT4	1.1 ± 0.78	0.6–1.15 ng/mL
TSH	2.03 ± 1.54	0.34–5.6 uIU/mL
Cortisol	250 ± 160	138–690 nmol/L
ACTH	17.8 ± 9.71	0–46 pg/mL
PRL	18.7 ± 18.9	M < 18 ng/mL; F < 24 ng/mL
GH (basal)	0.75 ± 1.08	0.06-5 ng/mL
GH (peak)	14.1 ± 13.91	> 16 ng/mlL
IGF-1	140.8 + 89.47	Specific age-gender limits

Table 3:

Urea	1.8–8.2 mmol/L
Potassium	3.5–5.0 mmol/L
Phosphate	0.8–1.4 mmol/L
Calcium	2.0–2.6 mmol/L
Creatinine	60–110 μmol/L (females)
	70–120 μmol/L (males)
Hemoglobin	120–140 g/L (females)
	140–160 g/L (males)
GFR	90–120 mL/min (1.5–2.0 mL/sec)

Table 4: Normal ranges of hormone

Hormone1	Normal Range
Testosterone	298 to 1,043 ng/dL
Free testosterone	3.5 to 17.9 ng/dL
DHT	31 to 193 ng/dL
DHT/T Ratio	0.052 to 0.33
DHT + T	372 to 1,349 ng/dL
SHBG	10.8 to 46.6 nmol/L
FSH	1.0 to 6.9 mIU/mL
LH	1.0 to 8.1 mIU/mL
E2	17.1 to 46.1 pg/mL

Table 5: Progesterone in pregnancy

When	Normal Values	What Level Means
Mid Luteal Phase	5+ ng/mL	As mentioned above, a level of 5 indicates some kind of ovulatory activity, though most doctors want to see a level over 10 on unmedicated cycles, and over 15 with medications. There is no mid-luteal level that predicts pregnancy
First Trimester	10–90 ng/ml	Average is about 20 at 4 weeks LMP, and 40 at 14 weeks LMP. It is important to note that while a higher progesterone level corresponds with higher pregnancy success rates, one cannot fully predict outcome based on progesterone levels. Progesterone supplementation is unlikely to help if started after a positive pregnancy test
Second Trimester	25–90 ng/mL	Average is 40 at beginning, 90 at end.
Third Trimester	49–423 ng/mL	Usually peaks at about 175.

Table 6: hCG levles in early pregnancy

Post Ovulation/Retrieval	Weeks/Days (LMP) Days	Average Singleton Level	Average Twin Level
10	3w3d	25	
12	3w5d	50	
14	4w0d	100	
16	4w2d	200	

Early-detection pregnancy tests (detecting 20 miu/mL hCG) can assist you in detecting pregnancy before your missed period.

Table 7: Oral glucose tolerance test for gestational diabetes

Time	Normal Values	
Fasting	< 150 mg/dL	Gestational diabetes is diagnosed if 2 or more levels are above the normal range. It is treated through diet, insulin injections, and sometimes with metformin. You may want to check all about gestational diabetes.
1 hour	< 190 mg/dL	
2 hours	< 165 mg/dL	
3 hours	< 145 mg/dL	

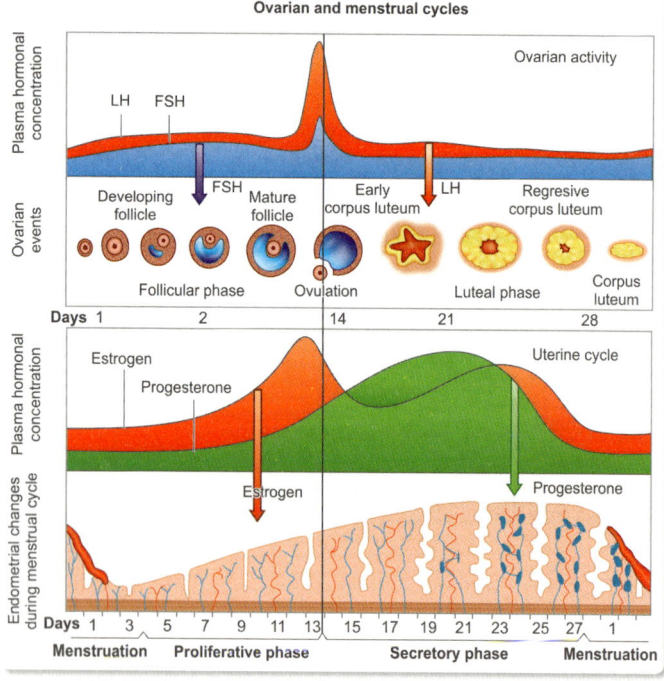

Fig. 1: Ovarian and menstrual cycles (For colour version see plate 8)

Table 8: Levels of various hormones in females

Hormone	Timing	Level	Notes
Follicle Stimulating Hormone (FSH)	Day 3	3–20 mIU/mL	FSH is often used as a gauge of ovarian reserve. In general, under 6 is excellent, 6-9 is good, 9-10 fair, 10-13 diminished reserve, 13+ very hard to stimulate. In PCOS testing, the LH:FSH ratio may be used in the diagnosis. The ratio is usually close to 1:1, but if the LH is higher, it is one possible indication of PCOS
Estradiol (E2)	Day 3	25–75 pg/mL	Levels on the lower end tend to be better for stimulating. Abnormally, high levels on day 3 may indicate existence of a functional cyst or diminished ovarian reserve
Estradiol (E2)	Day 4–5 of mods	100+ pg/mL or 2x Day 3	There are no charts showing E2 levels during stimulation since there is a wide variation depending on how many follicles are being produced and their size. Most doctors will consider any increase in E2 a positive sign, but others use a formula of either 100 pg/mL after 4 days of stims, or a doubling in E2 from the level taken on cycle day 3
Estradiol (E2)	Surge/hCG day	200+ pg/mL	The levels should be 200-600 per mature (18 mm) follicle. These levels are sometimes lower in overweight women

Contd...

Contd...

Luteinizing Hormone (LH)	Day 3	<7 mIU/mL	A normal LH level is similar to FSH. An LH that is higher than FSH is one indication of PCOS
Prolactin	Day 3	<24 ng/mL	Increased prolactin levels can interfere with ovulation. They may also indicate further testing (MRI) should be done to check for a pituitary tumor. Some women with PCOS also have hyperprolactinemia
Progesterone (P4)	Day 3	< 1.5 ng/mL	Often called the follicular phase level. An elevated level may indicate a lower pregnancy rate. If low progesterone levels are an issue for you, consider taking a natural fertility supplement
Progesterone (P4)	7 dpo	> 15 ng/mL	A progesterone test is done to confirm ovulation. When a follicle releases its egg. It becomes what is called a corpus luteum and produces progesterone. A level over 5 probably indicates some form of ovulation, but most doctors want to see a level over 10 on a natural cycle, and a level over 15 on a medicated cycle. There is no mid-luteal level that predicts pregnancy. Some say the test may be more accurate if done first thing in the morning after fasting

Contd...

Contd...

Thyroid Stimulating Hormone (TSH)	Day 3	0.4–4 uIU/ml	Mid-range normal in most labs is about 1.7. A high level of TSH combined with a low or normal T4 level generally indicates hypothyroidism, which can have an effect on fertility
Free Triiodothyronine (T3)	Day 3	1.4–4.4 pg/ml	Sometimes, the diseased thyroid gland will start producing very high levels of T3 but still produce normal levels of T4. Therefore, measurement of both hormones provides an even more accurate evaluation of thyroid function
Free Thyroxine (T4)	Day 3	0.8–2 ng/dL	A low level may indicate a diseased thyroid gland or may indicate a non-functioning pituitary gland, which is not stimulating the thyroid to produce T4. If the T4 is low and the TSH is normal, that is more likely to indicate a problem with the pituitary
Total Testosterone	Day 3	6–86 ng/dL	Testosterone is secreted from the adrenal gland and the ovaries. Most would consider a level above 50 to be somewhat elevated
Free Testosterone	Day 3	0.7–3.6 pg/mL	
Dehydroepiandrosterone Sulfate (DHEAS)	Day 3	35–430 ug/dL	An elevated DHEAS level may be improved through use of dexamethasone, prednisone, or insulin-sensitizing medications

Contd...

Contd...

Androstenedione	Day 3	0.7–3.1 ng/mL	
Sex Hormone Binding Globulin (SHBG)	Day 3	18–114 nmol/L	Increased androgen production often leads to lower SHBG
17 Hydroxy-progesterone	Day 3	20–100 ng/dL	Mid-cycle peak would be 100–250 ng/dL, luteal phases 100–500 ng/dL
Fasting Insulin	8–16 hours fasting	<30 mIU/mL	The normal range here doesn't give all the information. A fasting insulin of 10–13 generally indicates some insulin resistance, and levels above 13 indicate greater insulin resistance

Index

Page numbers followed by *f* refer to figure and *t* refer to table.

A

Andrology set up 47
    accessories used in 52*f*
Andrology work up 47
Antisperm antibodies 97
Arcuate uterus 100*f*
ART, complication of 116
Asherman's syndrome 15
Atrophic ovary 35*f*
Azoospermia 97

B

Blastocyst transfer 110

C

Calcium 120
Centrifuge machine 50*f*
Cervix and cervicitis 16*f*
Conception, pathway of 2, 2*f*
Congenital azoospermia, causes of 98
Creatinine 120

E

Echinacea purpura 5
Egg donation cycle 111
Embryo cryopreservation 111
Embryo development 72*f*
    and implantation 3, 3*f*
Embryo donation cycle 112
Embryo freezing 85, 111
    tools 86*f*
Embryo thawing 88
Embryo transfer 73*f*
    stimulation protocol for 74*f*
Embryos 73*f*
Embryoscope time lapse 76
Endometrial receptivity assay 80*f*
Endometrioma 37*f*
Endometriosis 40
    management of 40*f*
Epididymal sperm 66
External genitalia, of female 10*f*

F

Fallopian tube 13
Fasting insulin 126
Female evaluation and management 33
Female infertility, evaluation of 103
Female partner, workup of 31
Female reproductive system 10*f*
Fertilization 72*f*
    process 17*f*

Follicles and endometrium, color Doppler in 24f
Follicular growth and hormonal regulation 12f

G

Gestational diabetes, oral glucose tolerance test for 122t
Gestational surrogacy 112
Ginkgo biloba 5

H

Hemoglobin 120
    levels of 119t
Hormonal regulation, in females 13f
Hormone, normal ranges of 120t
Hormone level, in females 123t
Hypothalmus
Hysterosalpingography 15f

I

ICSI fertilization 72f
In vitro fertilization 108
Infertile couple 4
    management of 90, 92
    routine investigation of 31f
    special tests for 32f
Infertility 96
    approach to 4
    causes of 6
    factors in 6f
        control 1f
    in PCOS patients 117
    management, laparoscopic evaluation of 42f
    role in 96f
    tests for 30f, 105
    treatment 117
        complications of 80
    work-up, sequence of 17
Insemination, timing of 102f
Insemination/timed intercourse, stimulation protocol for 64f
Intrauterine insemination 64f, 100
    advantage of 101
IVF cycle, fertilization in 116
IVF, steps in 71, 71f
IVF/ICSI cycle 117

K

Kallmann's syndrome 11

L

Laparoscopy algorithm 42
Lapse embryo assesment 68
Luteal phase defect 44
  management of 44f
Luteinizing hormone 124

M

Male chromosome 67f
Male factor
    anatomical 7
    ejaculatory 6
    endocrine 9
    genetic 9

immunological infertility 8
infective 9
infertility 97
  evaluation of 45f
sperm 7
viscous semen 8
Male fertility 97
Male partner, workup of 45
Male reproductive system 7f
Male, female and idiopathic causes of infertility 4f
Male, hormonal circuit in 8f
Menstrual cycle 11f

O

Oligospermia 97
Oocytes 73f
Ovarian abnormality 15f
Ovarian and menstrual cycles 122f
Ovarian function treatment 35f
Ovarian hyperstimulation syndrome 110
Ovarian problems 35
Ovarian puncture 71f
Ovarian reserve 99
Ovarian stimulation
  antagonist protocol 70f
  long protocol 69f
  short protocol 69f
Ovarian tumor 37f
Ovary 34
  dermoid in 36f
  normal 34f
Ovulation cycle 34f
Ovulation detection kits 23f
Ovulation induction 39

Ovulation problem 38
Ovulation, management of 38f
Ovulation-stimulation agents 39f

P

Phosphate 120
Pituitary 13f
Polycystic ovary syndrome 14f, 36f, 107
Potassium 120
Pregnancy
  coitus affect 106
  hCG levles in early 121t
Preimplantation diagnosis 77f
Progesterone 124
  in pregnancy 121t

S

Semen analysis 18
  report 21f
Semen collection room 19f
Semen collection, protocol of 70f
Semen culture media 83f
Semen examination and processing 52
Semen extraction, evaluation and 97f
Semen freezing 81
  cryocans used for 85f
Semen fructose 60
Semen pH 57
  strip and measurement tool 54f
Semen processing 61, 62f
  swim-up method 61f

Semen viscosity 56
Seminal fluid analysis 29
Seminogram, abnormal 46, 46f
Sex hormone 126
Sexual dysfunction 16
Smoking, effect of 98
Sperm agglutination score 55f
Sperm, anatomy 96f
Sperm count
   low 20f
   normal 20f
Sperm counting chamber 20f
Sperm function test 56
Sperm meter (semen analysis chamber) 48, 48f
Sperm, morphology 58
Sperm retrieval techniques 66
Sperm transportation to uterine tube 51f
Sperm, vitality 57
Sperm warmer 49, 49f
Sperm, criteria of distinguishing 54f
Spermatogenesis in testis 9f
Spermatogenic process 96
Sperms, abnormal 20f
Swim up from pellet procedure 82f

T

Testes and seminal tract, pathology of 66f
Testicular biopsy 26, 67f
Testis, section of 7f
Thyroid stimulating hormone 125
Time lapse embryoscope 78f
Tubal abnormality 15f
Tubal factor 41
   of infertility management 41f

U

Urea 120
Uterine abnormality 15f
Uterotubal anomalies 103
Uterus 15

V

Varicocele, USG of 29f
Vitrified embryo on microtip 87f